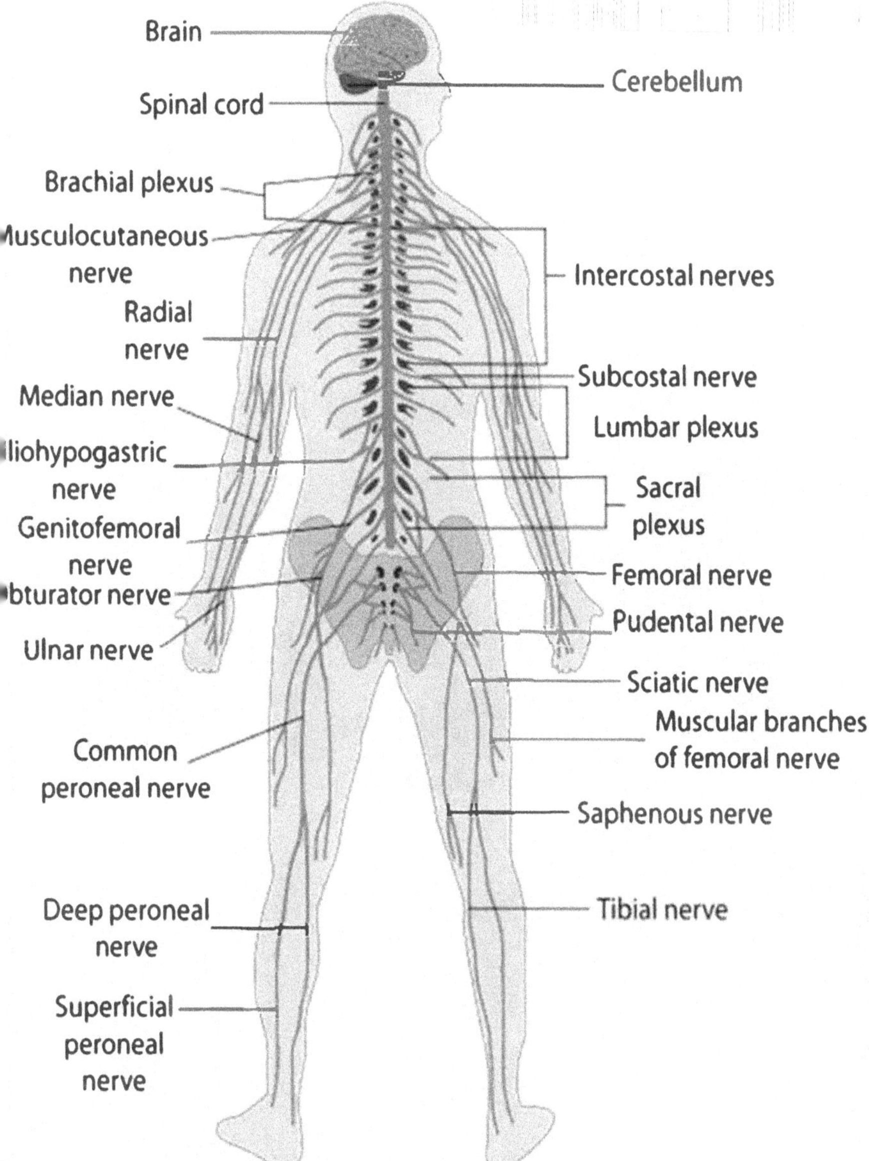

Brain
Cerebellum
Spinal cord
Brachial plexus
usculocutaneous nerve
Intercostal nerves
Radial nerve
Subcostal nerve
Median nerve
Lumbar plexus
liohypogastric nerve
Sacral plexus
Genitofemoral nerve
Femoral nerve
bturator nerve
Pudental nerve
Ulnar nerve
Sciatic nerve
Muscular branches of femoral nerve
Common peroneal nerve
Saphenous nerve
Tibial nerve
Deep peroneal nerve
Superficial peroneal nerve

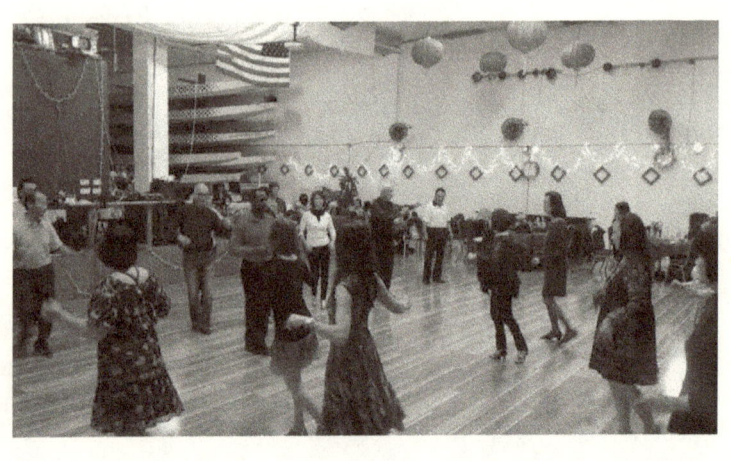

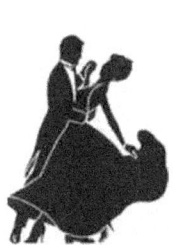

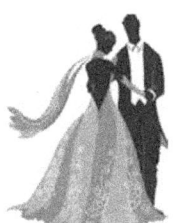

CHOREOLOGY BASIC

HEALING THROUGH DANCE

Elementary Smooth & Rhythm Syllabus!

Volume II

MICHEL F. JACQUES

Copyright © 2020 by Michel F. Jacques.

ISBN   978-1-970160-82-6 Ebook
ISBN   978-1-970160-83-3 Paperback

All rights reserved. No part of this publication may be reproduced, distributed, or transmitted in any form or by any means, including photocopying, recording, or other electronic or mechanical methods without the prior written permission of the publisher. For permission requests, solicit the publisher via the address below through mail or email with the subject line "Attention: Publication Permission".

The EC Publishing LLC books may be ordered
through booksellers or by contacting:

EC Publishing LLC
116 South Magnolia Ave.
Suite 3, Unit F
Ocala, FL 34471, USA
Direct Line: +1 (352) 644-6538
Fax: +1 (800) 483-1813
http://www.ecpublishingllc.com/
http://www.cidusa.org

Ordering Information:
Quantity sales. Special discounts are available on quantity purchases by corporations, associations, and others. For details, contact the publisher at the address above.

Printed in the United States of America

This book Choreology Basic Volume 2 is dedicated to my Three grown children: The late Bernard Felix Jacques, Stanley Jacques and Michelle PFindel Jacques. To my brothers and Sisters: Yves Gabriel Jacques, the Late Jean-Marie Robert Jacques, Charles Denis Jacques, Moise Antoine Jacques, Bernadin Maurice Jacques, Felix Bertin Jacques, Mireille Anne Louise Jacques, Yolande Laura Jacques, Maude Viviane Jacques, Josette Ketlie Jacques, Jude Forest Bataille, Rose Marie Saint-Paul, the late Thomas Saint-Paul.

To my Home School Teachers, my late mother Macilia Saint-Paul and my late father Emmanuel Ducamel Legagneur Jacques. To all my lovely best cousins, nieces and nephews. To all my mentors from Arthur Murray Dance Studio in Fort-Lauderdale, Pompano Beach, plantation, Sunrise. The late Mr. James Banta, to Brad & Cathie Lee Banta.

To my longtime coach the late Francois Szony and the late Toni Ann Gardella whom I have the honor to feature in the front cover of this book. I remember talking to him about this book 3 months before he passed away. But atlas, to all my Dance Partners, research colleagues and friends, Students and fans around the world

My joy knows no bounds in expressing my cordial gratitude to one of my best friend Olga Kane. Her keen interest in dancing and encouragement were a great help throughout the course of my research work. I humbly extend my thanks to all concerned colleagues and friends who co-operated with me in these regards.

It looks like yesterday when I landed to Miami airport From Port-au-Prince Haiti, July 27, 1984, in search of a better education. So, many Friends, professors, research companions and family members to mention. Hope you are enjoying reading it. Learning to dance well is like speaking a language fluently, the key to communication in a language fluently will lead the world to peace.

Your tax deductible $15 donation for a copy of this book will help dance educational, cultural after school program for children in Haiti and south Florida. Send a copy as a gift to a dear friend.

Order a copy through PayPal send to:
Hallandalesectioncid@gmail.com

Choreology Basic

Looking A this brain we can realize there are 4 parts we use as human. Those part will help us understand our perfect working simulator. What differentiate us from other species. I thought we were born with 60% human, 20% animal, 15% evil/hates and 5% spiritual giving us a total of 100% Brain capacity at birth.

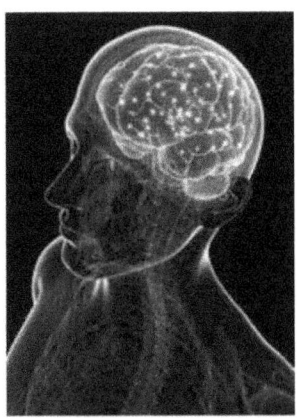

I did not want to recreate a brain simulator. My main goal was to conduct specific research study on the construction of human movements and the equivalence to music. For the past 35 years working in the realm of performing art, I view dancing as a cultural identity, a sacred and divine language that needed more attention when it comes to our children social, cultural, physical and mental wellbeing.

Experience proves that Dancing is a stimulator for the brain. Whatever we put in it, is exactly what we become. The brain proper function depends upon the communication between the cells in our body. The process of how thoughts are stored in our mind, is a highly complex study.

Dance instructors must continue doing research on many different forms of dance to compliment themselves. Because when we move from students to teachers, we would be able to follow the same principles. The fact is to train dancer to become entrepreneurs and entrepreneurs/leaders to become dance practitioners.

Many Dance instructors are teaching dancing based on their own vision, how they feel. So, many third world countries now are in the obligation to create a standardized system based on the 3 levels of their own cultural dance forms. Bronze, Silver and Gold to be part of the children social and cultural skills before they get to college.

In this book choreology basic volume 2, I am trying to be more realistic collecting data in biblical studies, ballroom and latin dancing to create a syllabus easier to follow steps to an ended result. This will allow our train instructors to interact and working together to differentiate between theoretical and experimental approaches.

Why do we enjoy listening to sad music? Research by frontiers

Sad music might actually evoke positive emotions reveals a new study by Japanese researchers published in the open-access journal *Frontiers in Psychology*. The findings help to explain why people enjoy listening to sad music, say Ai Kawakami and colleagues from Tokyo University of the Arts and the RIKEN Brain Science Institute, Japan.

Kawakami and colleagues asked 44 volunteers, including both musicians and non-specialists, to listen to two pieces of sad music and one piece of happy music. Each participant was required to use a set of keywords to rate both their perception of the music and their own emotional state.

The sad pieces of music included Glinka's "La Séparation" in F minor and Blumenfeld's Etude "Sur Mer" in G minor. The happy music piece was Granados's Allegro de Concierto in G major. To control for the "happy" effect of major key, they also played the minor-key pieces in major key, and vice versa.

The researchers explained that sad music evoked contradictory emotions because the participants of the study tended to feel sad music to be more tragic, less romantic, and less blithe than they felt themselves while listening to it.

"In general, sad music induces sadness in listeners, and sadness is regarded as an unpleasant emotion. If sad music actually evokes only unpleasant emotion, we would not listen to it," the researchers wrote in the study.

"Music that is perceived as sad actually induces romantic emotion as well as sad emotion. And people, regardless of their musical training, experience this ambivalent emotion to listen to the sad music," added the researchers.

Also, unlike sadness in daily life, sadness experienced through art actually feels pleasant, possibly because the latter does not pose an actual threat to our safety. This could help people to deal with their negative emotions in daily life, concluded the authors.

"Emotion experienced by music has no direct danger or harm unlike the emotion experienced in everyday life. Therefore, we can even enjoy unpleasant emotion such as sadness. If we suffer from unpleasant emotion evoked through daily life, sad music might be helpful to alleviate negative emotion," they added.

Dr. Sharpley Hsieh and colleagues from Neuroscience Research Australia (NeuRA) found that people with semantic dementia, a disease where parts of the left hemisphere are severely affected, have difficulty recognizing emotion in music.

These findings have exciting implications for our understanding of how music, language and emotions are handled by the brain.

"It's known that processing whether a face is happy or sad is impaired in people who lose key regions of the right hemisphere, as happens in people with Alzheimer's and semantic dementia", says Dr. Hsieh.

"What we have now learnt from looking at people with semantic dementia is that understanding emotions in music involves key parts of the other side of the brain as well", she says.

"Ours is the first study from patients with dementia to show that language-based areas of the brain, primarily on the left, are important for extracting <u>emotional</u> meaning from music. Our findings suggest that the brain considers melodies and speech to be similar and that overlapping parts of the brain are required for both", says Hsieh.

This paper is published in the journal Neuropsychologia.

According to the publishers journal neuropsychology. People with Alzheimer's disease lose episodic memory ('What did I do yesterday?'); people with semantic dementia lose semantic memory ('What is a zebra?'). Dr. Hsieh studied people with Alzheimer's disease, semantic dementia and healthy people without either disease. Participants were played new pieces of music and had to indicate whether the song was happy, sad, peaceful or scary.

- Images were then taken of the patients' brains using MRI so that diseased parts of the brain could be compared statistically to the answers provided in the musical test.

- Patients with Alzheimer's and semantic dementia have problems deciding whether a human face looks happy or sad because the amygdala in the right hemisphere is diseased.

- Patients with semantic <u>dementia</u> have additional problems labelling whether a piece of music is happy or sad because the anterior temporal lobe in the left hemisphere is diseased.

I want to take the opportunity to share with my colleagues and friends readers of this volume choreology basic, the research study based on the theory of the origin of dance. Brought to me by one of my colleagues associate Mr. Ristic Steven an active Member of CID-Unesco at our 3rd congress on dance research in Hallandale beach.

We live at the moment in time of Hi-Tech civilization and Hi-Democratic society which is based on achievement of industrial and technology revolution, meaning on revolutionary discoveries of steam machine and automatic swaddling machine, what is brought it to appearance of enormous surplus of the free time. Working time has drastically reduced

Choreology Basic

on all level, and even lower layers of society had opportunity to be a part of any kind of social life. If we look strictly for and about the dance, that was the time when also and common people had a opportunity to begin to dance, meaning practice of dance as well as creating, researching and think about it. Before that time, logically thinking and analyzing, dance belonged to layers of people who had enough free time for fun, and who had a need for all kind of entertainment. Also logically thinking and analyzing, we told about nobility and them who work for nobility, better says, them who were paid to entertain nobility. And, going further with this direction, but this time we will consider social sciences, we can said that parallel with industrial revolution we had a beginning of ruining of, till that, traditional social order characteristic for Middle Age, based on division of society on:

- Nobility, or landowners

- Serfs, or them who works on land

- Middle class, who lived in cities, meaning of tradespeople, clergy and all others „free" people, but without much freedom in full sense of that word

Of course, there we talk about French bourgeois revolution which was almost parallel with English industrial revolution. And, since then, beside of dance, also other categories of art were accessible for all layers of society. Also, we can say, and education and science were freed from nobilities and clergies chains, and that was time of beginning of, as we said before, entrance of dance in all layers of society, but also and beginning of research of dance, and we had a plenty of theories, books and others ways of presentation of knowledge about of the dance. So, considering about that, may intense is to present all of that what was before of that period, especially beginning of dance, or moment when the dance begin to be a cultural category, not just unconsciously and unduly movements and steps.

One of the important chapter of that book it shall be, for example, my try to described relationship between dance and religions, and then we will explain more of that period, from the earliest ancient religions till the emergency of Christianity, and, also important, emergency of Judaism, Hinduism, Buddhism, Islam and all others existing religion. We will try to prove that in one moment of history, dance became a great danger for religions and very small numbers of religions use dance like a part of religious service. Also, after the English Industrial and French Bourgeois Revolutions, things became to change. Of course, if we don't mentioned others religions, that doesn't mean that that religions had a smaller influence in developing a dance like a cultural category, on the contrary, in chapter about relationship dance and religion we will explained all existing and ancients religions important and connected with dance in all forms.

Also, we must say that nations we will mention here is not a nation in today's sense, because, as the today's science said, we can talk about nations just from 19-th centuries, which is also connect with revolutions we mentioned before. In many ways, before, religions, states and official politics didn't recognize dance as the elite and noble art, for many reasons, and we will explain that.

But, we will see, dance remains in many ways similar as it was in beginning, and, if we know important facts, it is relatively easy to follow main characteristics of dance from beginning till now. So we can say that dance changed as well as mankind, in some ways dance was and before his own time, and, knowing the some other facts from anthropology, sociology, ethnology and philosophy from which they came about, we can say that is one of the reason why dance not was recognized in properly way. Of course, it shall be explained more in chapter dedicated to that.

And last, but not least, and also connected with nations, but also with many other things, we must emphasize that we will present theme by the principles and methods of philosophy of dance founded by Dr. Alkis Raftis which allows us to see and other side of things, not just in straight line like permits us a mainstream science. Also, we shall use all advantages and methods of community studies, one of the latest science, and let us say more in that way, anthropology is science about the individuals, sociology is science about the society, and that, community science is study a relations between individuals and groups in community, or, we will study a group developing theory starting from ideas about a dancers as the members of same or different groups. Let's say that in more romantic way,

Choreology Basic

we will not look down to find a facts about the dance, like archeologist work, to research a dance we will lift head to the sky, particularly, as we will prove, in the night sky what is in many ways important for theory of dance!

"at first there was a step"-

I was thinking a lot what and how much word I shall use for this my attempt to make allusion on Holly Bible. My dilemma it was: movement, step, or maybe both? At the end I choose just a step because the movement is something that had also and animals and plants, but in many sciences we told about differences from that moment when the first man was up, or, since appearance of Homo erectus and Homo sapiens. That's mean, step is great advantage what our ancestors did in the way of separating from animals and creating something that today we call a mankind.

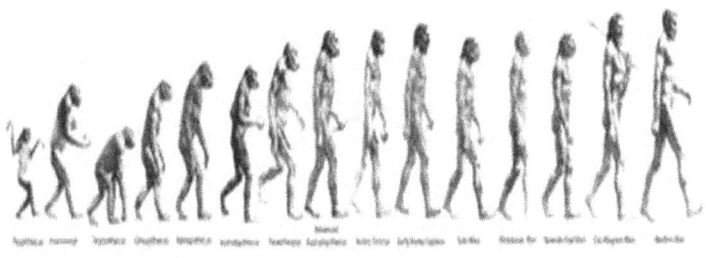

Further In that direction, we will follow way of thinking that our ancestors, or, maybe better to say, we will monitor the development of their needs till the moments when we can talk the step was transformed to something we can call dance. And more further, maybe we can say that erecting is one of the condition who bring to the beginning of thinking process, and that's mean that when the man began to think, that is time when the movement began to be a step. And, first result of thinking was that man began to think about his needs. To better understanding of that we talk about first must to understand a development of human needs. In the earlier time we told about 3 basic needs, primary, secondary and tertiary but in last time, thanks to American psychologist Abraham Maslow we can say that also and need for non-material things is very important for our story and, of course, for development of mankind, especially if we are focused in origin and development of dance. So, there is one of the simplest examples of Maslow's pyramid:

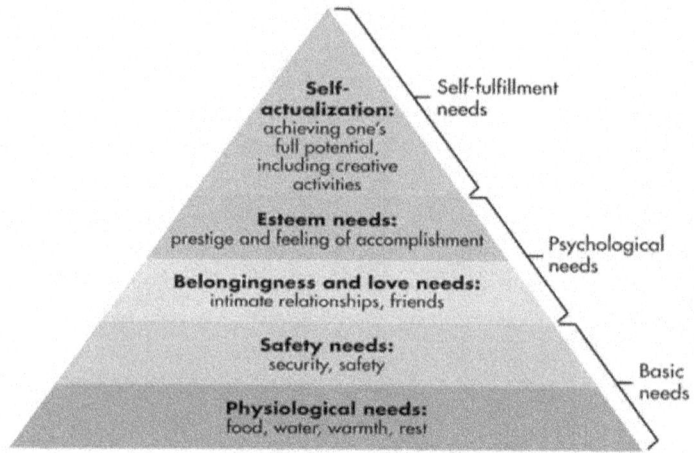

And, based on that we will analyze, through the time, development of step and when and why it became a dance.

As we see in pyramid, on the base is just physiological needs, and it is logic to think that it was took through the longest period to fit completely how to satisfy and to be conscious of that needs, and that it was basic prerequisite to move to a higher level of thinking about solving the problems.

There we will try to focus just on that what is important for dance, meaning, to not to interfere in other areas of science, we will follow just a step. That's mean, we will analyze just step developing and influence that step made in process of thinking, trying to put ourselves in the position of the then man. But we must say that step was first departure and separate from animals, and main reason why men straighten up was, in fact, his trying to ease fulfilling they needs. Following that logic, we can say when the men facilitate satisfying needs, in this period of developing they made another needs, and, at the end, when the circle was closed in some way, from that kind of primitive thinking, and finding ways to make it easier to meet your needs can became a kind of needs. In the same ways, we can call that a beginning of creative thinking, but also a try to fulfill a free time, or, simpler, maybe that is time when we can talk about appearance a need for fun!

Choreology Basic

Later we will elaborate more about that, now let's start with a step and how many steps in dancing we know? Under the term step first association for all of us is step how we walk. But we need to put ourselves in position of Homo sapiens 200,000 years from now, and to ask ourselves what was first purpose of step? Maybe the first step was run, because first purpose of step was to run away from possible enemy? Or, maybe, purpose could be to catch the spoil, in the beginning of his hunting career? But, if we talk about the hunting, so that step had to be connected with the jump. So, till now, we mentioned 3 types of steps:

1- Walking step

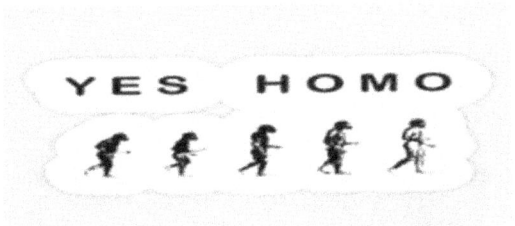

2- Running step

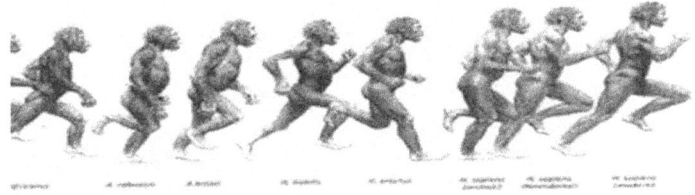

3- Jumping step

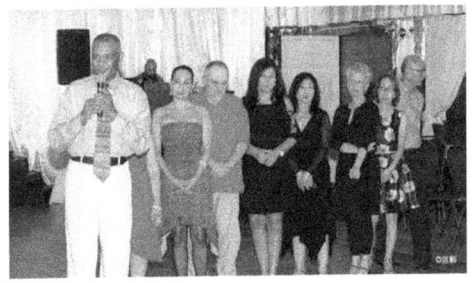

Michel F. Jacques

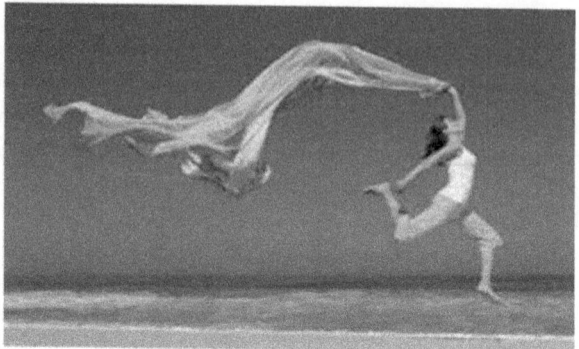

and, we couldn't tell exactly what is oldest, but, we can say that is what all types of steps was, in a sociological sense, just a mean to meet the physiological needs, and, there I want to emphasize one movement which we also call step, and which is maybe most important element for our story of dance, in same time probably and oldest.

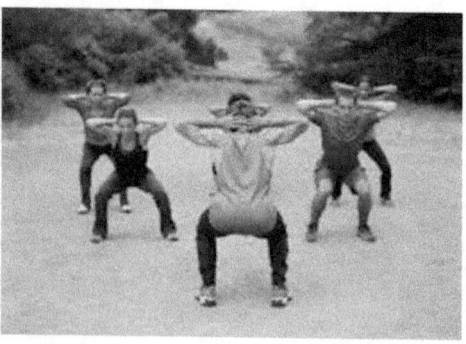

Maybe we can say on better way, let's try to find the answer little lower, so, story of the squat follows, and first question which we will ask it shell be, is the squat step? According to the valid and current dance theories – step is every movement which in any way disturbs of balance – we can say that squat is step also. Looking at the sociological standpoint, we can say that squat had a very important role in developing processes of thinking and raising awareness, much more than other kinds of step, and, based on that fact, we can freely say that the squat is oldest step. Of course, we will not mentioned which physiological need we most easily meet by squatting, but, proof of what we have said before about importance of squat, shall be fact that when we are in position of squatting the concentration increase, and surely that has led it to the some kind of primitive thinking, and further to the development of aware of the possibilities of using and other kinds of step to meet the other needs. So, that's mean, from a four-legged to a upright position sure we came through the position of squatting, and, by the step theory we proved that squat is step, and in many ways we can say that squat is first and most important step which plays a very important role in transforming steps in the dance. The vitality of the squat can be demonstrated by the fact that it is still an important and very alive element of many dances all over the world, for example, Russian dances.

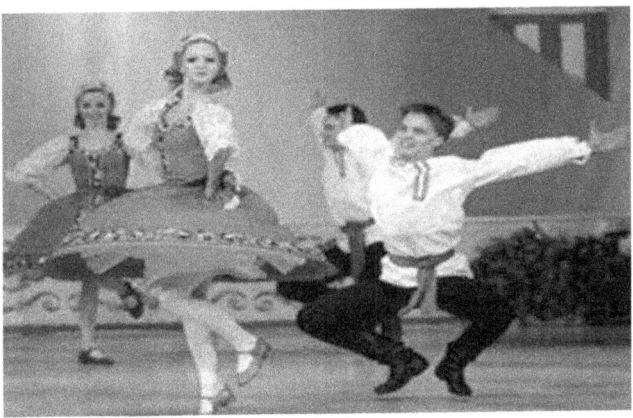

Of course, at the moment we talk in text about squat as step, which was transformed later in dance element, and remain until today. And, last but not least in first chapter, we have to point up a time distance from today, and that period is very large. Archeology and anthropology teach us that the Homo sapiens exist from before 200 000 years, that's mean, if we look carefully and logic on Maslow's phyramid, we can conclude that the phase of satisfying only physiological needs lasted not less than 100 000 years. Next level, when beside the physiological, satisfied and first psychological needs, in proportion as say Maslow, should have lasted about 50 000-60 000 years. And further, next level about 20 000-25 000 years, than 10 000-15 000 years, at the end, top level when we could say that step became a dance, was about 5 000 years ago, and, that's mean that thinking through how to best meet his needs led to acceleration of new

Michel F. Jacques

discoveries, but, one more time to emphasize, we are investigating strictly dance and all about dancing, and we will keep stick to that principle. Also, we can see that and today all that kind of steps is very important elements of the dance, and now, can we exactly say when the step became a dance?

Research made by Prof. Ristic Stevan

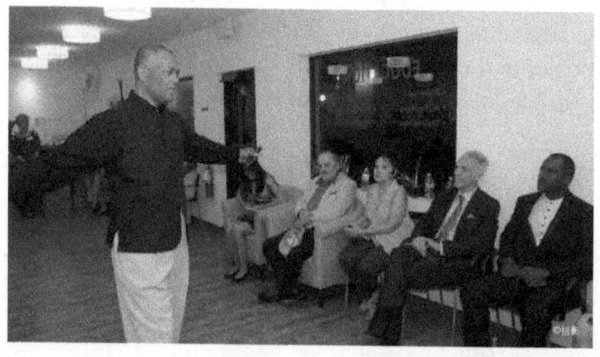

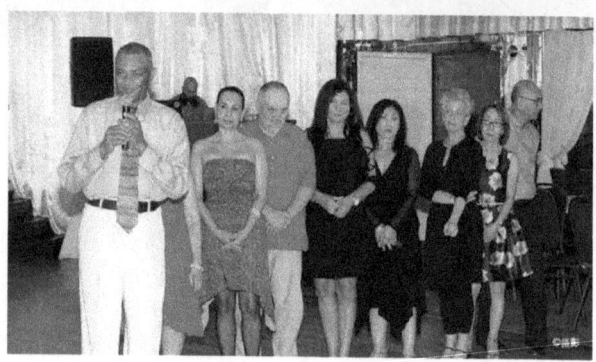

If you search the Global Dance Directory using "therapy" as keyword you get 2600 listings. This means that approximately one in every hundred dance professionals provides some form of therapy. Though 0.01% is a very small percentage, therapy is probably the most rapidly expanding branch of the dance industry. The proliferation of courses and workshops shows that the number of dance therapists has the potential to double every year. Qualified professionals are increasingly employed in hospitals, health centers, aged persons' homes, prisons or mental asylums. Private practices are multiplying, and so are conventional dance schools offering therapy classes.

This boom might be due to the fact that curing through dance comes under the Ministry of Health in many countries, so the possibility of funding is incomparably higher than when dance is oriented towards performance or recreation. Another reason is that, since our modern way of life has alienated man from primary functions, people are rediscovering the power of dance to heal.

Dancing certainly makes a healthy person feel better but seeking to alleviate a manifest psychological problem through dance is another thing. Traditional societies have preserved well-being by providing frequent opportunities to dance in social gatherings and in rituals. Since these events have been abandoned our frustration has accumulated, so now we turn to sessions by professionals to satisfy that need. Specific dances have been used to cure some illnesses - research is required to find out if those dances can be used today for the same purpose.

Even more impressive is the fact that patients have been cured not by their own dancing but by the dancing of another person. In many countries of the world people ask healers, shamans and witchdoctors called voodoo priest to continue age-old practices because they find them beneficial. These dances, rejected so far by industrialized societies, deserve serious study.

> What I want to do is to share these research studies of Music & Dance with the coming generations. Music & dance are special Languages, and music and dance together can communication things that are difficult to communicate with words. Specially things that are related to emotion we, must share as human being. There is always and forever the joy in the music and the dance.

Michel F. Jacques

Dancing can reverse the signs of aging in the brain

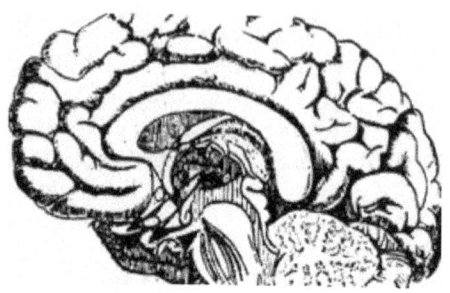

Credit to CC0 Public Domain

As we grow older we suffer a decline in mental and physical fitness, which can be made worse by conditions like Alzheimer's disease. A new study, published in the open-access journal *Frontiers in Human Neuroscience*, shows that older people who routinely partake in physical exercise can reverse the signs of aging in the brain, and dancing has the most profound effect.

"Exercise has the beneficial effect of slowing down or even counteracting age-related decline in mental and physical capacity," says Dr Kathrin Rehfeld, lead author of the study, based at the German center for Neurodegenerative Diseases, Magdeburg, Germany. «In this study, we show that two different types of physical exercise (dancing and endurance training) both increase the area of the brain that declines with age. In comparison, it was only dancing that lead to noticeable behavioral changes in terms of improved balance.»

Elderly volunteers, with an average age of 68, were recruited to the study and assigned either an eighteen-month weekly course of learning dance routines, or endurance and flexibility training. Both groups showed an increase in the hippocampus region of the brain. This is important because this area can be prone to age-related Decline and is affected by diseases like Alzheimer›s. It also plays a key role in memory and learning, as well as keeping one›s balance.

While previous research has shown that Physical exercise combat age-related brain decline, it is not known if one type of exercise can be better than another. To assess this, the exercise routines given to the volunteers differed. The traditional fitness training program conducted mainly repetitive exercises, such as cycling or Nordic walking, but the dance group were challenged with something new each week.

Dr Rehfeld explains, "We tried to provide our seniors in the dance group with constantly changing dance routines of different genres (Jazz, Square, Latin-American and Line Dance). Steps, arm-patterns, formations, speed and rhythms were changed every second week to keep them in a constant learning process. The most challenging aspect for them was to recall the routines under the pressure of time and without any cues from the instructor.

These extra challenges are thought to account for the noticeable difference in balance displayed by those participants in dancing group. Dr Rehfeld and her colleagues are building on this research to trial new fitness programs that have the potential of maximizing anti-aging effects on the brain.

"Right now, we are evaluating a new system called "Jymmin" (jamming and gymnastic). This is a sensor-based system which generates sounds (melodies, rhythm) based on physical activity. We know that dementia patients react strongly when listening to music. We want to combine the promising aspects of physical activity and active music making in a feasibility study with dementia patients."

Dr Rehfeld concludes with advice that could get us up out of our seats and dancing to our favorite beat.

"I believe that everybody would like to live an independent and healthy life, for as long as possible. Physical activity is one of the lifestyle factors that can contribute to this, counteracting several risk factors and slowing down age-related decline. I think dancing is a powerful tool to set new challenges for body and mind, especially in older age.»

This study falls into a broader collection of research investigating the <u>cognitive and neural effects of physical and cognitive activity across the lifespan</u>. Brain imaging reveals how neural responses to different types of music really affect the emotion regulation of persons. The study concludes that men who process negative feelings with music react negatively to aggressive and sad music.

Emotion regulation is an essential component to <u>mental health</u>. Poor <u>emotion regulation</u> is associated with psychiatric mood disorders such as depression. Clinical <u>music</u> therapists know the power music can have over emotions, and are able to use music to help their clients to better mood states and even to help relieve symptoms of psychiatric mood disorders like depression. But many people also listen to music on their own as a means of emotion regulation, and not much is known about how this kind of music listening affects mental health. Researchers at the Centre for Interdisciplinary Music Research at the University of Jyväskylä, Aalto University in Finland and Aarhus University in Denmark decided to investigate the relationship between mental health, music listening habits and neural responses to music emotions by looking at a combination of behavioural and neuroimaging data. The study was published in August in the journal *Frontiers in Human Neuroscience*.

"Some ways of coping with negative emotion, such as rumination, which means continually thinking over negative things, are linked to poor mental health. We wanted to learn whether there could be similar negative effects of some styles of music listening," explains Emily Carlson, a music therapist and the main author of the study. "We hope our research encourages music therapists to talk with their clients about their music use outside the session," concludes Emily Carlson, "and encourages everyone to think about the how the different ways they use music might help or harm their own well-being.

CID-UNESCO World Congress on Dance Research is being held in USA since 2015. Below is a report of the 4th annual international congress held in Hallandale Beach, Florida USA. November 2018.

The board of organizers and conferees deserve praise for all their hard work & contributions.

All participants at the Congress agreed that the Congress was very successful in all aspects, plus it brought to light some new ideas that appear to be very useful as a guide for the further work of CID or other dance organizations. During those four days we encountered some difficulties too, but it was all successfully resolved due to good teamwork. Just like every dance research congress, this year's congress consisted of three forms of presentation:

We can conclude that it was a very successful Congress. It was a platform where participants managed to answer some very important questions about the current state of the dance world and to point out possible problems that may occur within dance community.

I am not going to list all the names and countries of all participants in this report, but I will simply summarize main conclusions of some workshops and I will emphasize the importance of the informal conversations during free time and while socializing after the formal workshops and presentations. These conclusions can be divided into three basic directions, namely:

1. The need to move to a higher level of education on the theory of dance
2. To emphasize the importance of ballroom dance exercise therapy and other forms of treatment with the use of dance
3. The need for a better organization within dance community in order to protect interests of our communities.

1. Education

The problem with dance education is mostly related to North America, however, this does not mean, in any way, that Europe has a satisfactory dance educational system. As far as the USA is concerned, the biggest problem is the lack of adequate materials for studying the background and the history of the dance. So, we often see a situation where choreographers, dance teachers and dancers need to focus their creative energy on research and theoretical proof to justify their ideas instead of concentrating on implementation of their creative ideas.

It is therefore agreed that a unique textbook shall be written, and it should be used in all dance schools and other dance institutions at all levels and for all types of dances. Particular attention should be paid to the latest discoveries in the field of dance research. In particular, it is important to support, in all possible ways, the visits of as many CID members from the USA to congresses in Europe and to bring as many members from Europe to congresses in USA; members of CID who have potentials to change the current situation by providing needed education materials.

It is also necessary to change the mindset of dividing the dance culture into several levels, i.e. ballet and related dances are considered as *elite* forms, while so-called entertainment dances are lower dance forms.

A confirmation of disadvantages of such divisions can be seen in other fields of art, however we can see advantages when we change current mindset. An example is this year's Nobel Prize for Literature, awarded to Bob Dylan. This award proved that rock-poetry is of the same importance as poetry of Yesenin, for example. Similarly, a parallel can be drawn if we look at Tango Argentinian and think of it as an equal part of the culture as the Swan Lake is.

2. Dance-Therapy

Particularly good results are seen in the field of dance therapy and other forms of healing where dance is used as a primary or secondary instrument. It is important to mention an excellent lecture by Dr. Lynn Migdal, which included all the experiences of the dance-therapy principles so far. Her lecture also showed in which direction this area of work should be further developed.

Choreology Basic

The most important thing in her lecture was a connection between good theoretical background and perfect practical application when treating specific disease. She also showed some successful implementation of new revolutionary ideas that we hope to see in the future proved to be valid and correct. We are talking about the introduction of the concept of "Breathing as a form of dance". This concept highlights the power of action-oriented concentration on the unconscious workings of the human body. Justifiably, we can ask whether this exercise could be used to try to control the heartbeat?

We know that there are witnesses and records that some Yoga masters in Tibet have done this successfully, although this is not scientifically proven, this is certainly the direction in which we can steer further research.

It is especially interesting to observe the differences in dance-therapy in America, Europe and Russia. In Europe folk dance is most commonly used as a basic instrument in therapy, in Russia ballet, while in the USA most commonly used form of dance is ballroom dance. This is completely understandable, and it underlines the fact that all dances are of equal importance for dance therapy. A conclusion and recommendation of this congress is that even basics of Indian and Chinese dance traditions should be included in the development of dance therapy.

The problem that remains is the insufficient exploration of Africa and some other areas. It was agreed to start researches of those areas in 2018 and 2019. Once we complete the research, we hope to include those dance forms in the concept of dance therapy. This is important because of the presence of these cultures in US dance life, and because we can see basic dance elements of these cultures in the dance tradition of the USA and Latin America.

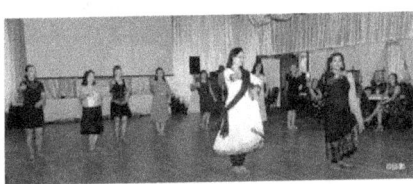
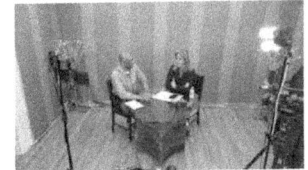

Michel F. Jacques

4. Stage performances

This form of presentation was, as expected, the most impressive at the congress, which once again, demonstrated the correctness, stability and quality of American principles of education and presentation of dance. There were many attractive and interesting performances that showed a high level of creativity, enthusiasm and experience. Despite numerous great artists and dance works, we still must face the evidence that when it comes to the entertainment world, general opinion is that dance forms are quite neglected.

Especially if we look at film or music, we see a difference in profit, approaches, professionalism and overall treatment by other artists. Therefore, one of the conclusions of the congress is that that all those involved in dance art should be more unified, the congress recommendation is to do so under the aegis of the CID. This way dance artists can play a greater role in the Entertainment Industry, as well as to increase their earning.

I will make a parallel to Bob Dylan`s Nobel Prize again, so apart from a larger share of resources, we should also strive to create equality awareness, give the same importance to ballet, ballroom dancing and all other kinds of dance. We are not suggesting this just so other types of dance can equalized with ballet in the cultural sense. We are also considering more efficient way to include ballet in Entertainment Industry, so that artists involved in this form of dance can easier access necessary funds for their work.

A conclusion is that this Congress proved the constant progress of the dance in all its forms. During the congress we pointed out some obstacles and problems in the dance world too, but we also saw many ways of solving them out.

Many thanks, once again, to the organizer! We can freely say that main goals of the 3rd International Dance Research Congress have been achieved. The congress was a success and everyone who participated expressed their wish to come again year after…

Choreology Basic

SUMMARY of the Hallandale Section of Cid UNESCO.

This small organization is carrying forth a global vision to share the cultural, health and healing properties of organized dance to people everywhere. The International Congress is a large event which encompasses many aspects of dance education and has the capacity to act as the central organizing event for the organization. The idea of this big vision is gaining traction in South Florida and expanding nationally through certified dance instructors taking the programs out. The generosity and passion of the director, board and volunteers have made all of this happen in just a few years. Participants agreed it is time to take the organization to the next level and finances are the main barrier to this growth. Routine administrative tasks should be divided and delegated in order for the director to focus on capacity and fund development. It is important for the board of directors to fully understand the legal and fiduciary responsibilities they must fulfill on an annual budget. The structure of Hallandale CID needs to be aligned with an American 501C3 on reporting and financial management. In anticipating a growing budget, synchronizing these two structures will make reporting to all donors, the IRS and the CID much smoother. Expanding the board and leadership opportunities will go far in building capacity at the board and volunteer levels. The more organizational representatives who feel "ownership" of the mission will create strong advocates for marketing, fundraising and organizational sustainability. With a three-tiered mission of local, national and global impact, each area of focus will require professional capacity to manage and grow programs. Efforts to document past years financials and program growth will serve to build a financial platform for the consistent fundraising and grant writing that will be required for sustainability. Combined with current impact statements, Hallandale CID is well positioned to move forward with high growth to match their vision. A group of people committed to cultural continuity can achieve many things together. The passion in this organization is palpable and to be commended. Good luck in all of your future efforts.

HALLaNDALE SECTION CID 12/18 PAMELA KINGFISHER, SHINING WATERS CONSULTING

Michel F. Jacques

Lifecycles Placement Chart: The participants agreed that the organization is just moving into the growth stage with financial, administrative systems and governance not as well developed as necessary.

THE GROWTH STAGE Becoming Who You Are Overview: Program opportunity and service demand exceed current systems and structural capacities

Characteristics: • Program: Organization begins to understand and define the distinctive methods and approach that separate its programming from others • Management: Organization is led by people who see infinite potential for services • Governance: Board structure begins to appear • Resources: More sources of income create greater accounting and compliance complexities • Systems: Current systems, never good to begin with, must now be substantially improved to meet demands of continual program expansion and rising compliance expectations Challenges of the Growth Stage: • Too much to do, too little time • Developing board ownership • Creating a program and strategic focus that doesn't trap creativity and vision Management and leadership needs

• Dynamic • Strong base of personal reserves • Able to inspire and motivate • Energetic • Able to create a plan and provide focus, but veer from it as necessary • Able to appreciate, create and routinize systems to make certain functions easier • Good judgment and instinct to know what opportunities to pursue and which to decline • Comfortable with continual change

CRITICAL ISSUES 1. Governance: The board of directors should focus on annual duties of governance, such as policies and procedure updates, learning and implementing their fiduciary responsibilities regarding financial oversight. It will be important for the board to learn and implement financial management systems together, so the exercise becomes a routine administrative board activity. Assigning a "parliamentarian" role to the board vice president or secretary could ensure it is someone's duty to understand the IRS rules and nonprofit guidelines to assist in board decision making.

2. Marketing and Recruitment: The goal is to gain more recognition for the organization and individual programs in order to attract more volunteers, sponsors and audiences. It will be important to better articulate the local and global partnership in a succinct explanation for anyone to share. The updated website is a great portal into the organization, but it is time to initiate free social media such as Face Book and Instagram accounts, and assign a volunteer to run them.

3. Fundraising: Currently, leadership is seeking a contract grant writer but should continue to learn as a board together in order to manage a consultant, make strategic decisions and/or step in as needed. The board should continue to define donor and sponsorship opportunities for various programs in the community. Create "scripts" or one sheets for board and volunteers to utilize regarding each program to make asking for donations easier. The board of directors are the "ambassadors" of the organization and should actively assist in donor and sponsorship solicitation.

HALLANDALE SECTION CID 12/18 PAMELA KINGFISHER, SHINING WATERS CONSULTING

Document volunteer hours and calculate the "giving" numbers to prove in-kind support and to further understand the true cost of events and programs
SYSTEMS Financial: Spreadsheets may still be the easiest system for now, but as new grants and school contracts are obtained, leadership should explore purchasing QuickBooks for Nonprofits software for financial management. The organization utilizes a certified public accountant for IRS filings, but much of the financial management can be taken care of in-house as administrative staff is brought on. Future Needs: Research financial software for financial management Approve the budget at the beginning of the year and check in periodically to adjust

Administrative: The organization does not have its' own infrastructure at this time but relies on the founder's generosity. This is not a sustainable model for an organization with such a broad mission that includes programming that is local, national and international. Future Needs:

Formalizing staff positions with job descriptions with a budget forecast for hiring and maintaining staff Shared electronic platforms to coordinate board and international communications Determine which tasks can be shifted from the director

Development There are no systems in place for donor management and fundraising on a consistent basis. This work should be divided between director and board or a dedicated volunteer to manage the research of sponsors, donors and foundations. Utilizing this first Broward County grant to leverage other foundations and/or grants is important – don't miss this opportunity to build support. Future Needs: Fundraising training focusing on three areas of Sponsors, Donors and Foundation grants Create a development committee to take on the task of initiating a development plan for high growth Consider purchasing Donor software to manage multiple development efforts.

Marketing

The website is professional and inviting and seems to have the capacity to serve as a global platform for collected resources and communications. It is time to engage social media platforms as essential free marketing. Future Needs: Engage and utilize social media platforms Reach out to radio and print outlets with packages and event notices Press releases should be regularly utilized to consistently approach print media.

HALLANDALE SECTION CID 12/18 PAMELA KINGFISHER, SHINING WATERS CONSULTING

The organizations' Annual Dance Congress is led by a committee to oversee the planning and execution of such a big international event. It would be useful for any program committee to document measurable data on every event for evaluative and "case-making" processes. Documented evaluative information is important for continual assessment, budget review, time management and sharing program information with more people. Annual board meetings should reflect the reports on event production costs, revenue, attendance, volunteers, etc.

Future Needs: Design a fundraising plan to meet the annual budget; begin each year with a budget and a stretch goal Document program information (evaluative data) for the board and ongoing marketing efforts Continue to seek training for more board members and volunteers in grant writing and donor solicitations Develop systems for tracking all fundraising activities – this might be better organized by a committee.

GOVERNANCE - BOARD OF DIRECTORS

There are currently five board members serving the organization, but it was unclear to participants what their bylaws define for numbers of board members. It will be important for the board to be familiar with the bylaws to ensure they are fulfilling their obligations and following their rules. The CID Hallandale Board members are business professionals who understand sound financial management and transparency. The board meets monthly to discuss all matters related to planning, management, and implementation of policies. All records are stored at the office of the founder.

Future Needs: Recruit additional board members with specific skills needed for capacity building and growth Consider engaging younger people into committees or board leadership positions Review and update the bylaws on an annual basis during a board meeting Assign tasks to the four required board meetings per year (approve next year's budget; fundraising plan; mid-year program and budget evaluation; end of year review, evaluation and Learn the legalities of a U.S. based nonprofit organization in order to remain in compliance as an organization (as the international policies of a UNESCO chapter are well understood)

FINANCIAL POSITION The organization has been operating primarily with private income of the board, along with the use of office and studio space donated by Mr. Jacques. In order for the organization to grow and become sustainable, funding must be secured to establish a home office with administrative staff. Participants agreed it is time to grow into this next organizational phase.

Michel F. Jacques

The participants are very encouraged about fundraising and growing the annual budget. Working with the grant from Broward County Cultural Division is the first grant they will learn to manage and complete. They feel this grant opportunity "changes everything" in the organizations' trajectory and feel ready to step up and meet the responsibilities of meeting an annual budget.

Until now, CID Hallandale section relies mainly on volunteers, in-kind services and board generosity, but participants are ready to engage in future fundraising and grant writing.

Future Needs: Board members (or a committee) should seek out grant writing workshops and other opportunities to learn about fundraising techniques Establish fundraising "scripts" and packages for each program – these can be used to train each other and new volunteers to ask for donations, services or sponsorships

HALLANDALE SECTION CID 12/18 PAMELA KINGFISHER, SHINING WATERS CONSULTING

Hallandale CID utilizes International qualifications for dance instructors to be certified at the international level. In 2015, eight teachers graduated the certification program, which is a system to teach American dance styles, the English language, as well as American music to an International audience.

Currently, Hallandale CID chapter organizes at least ten annual events each year including lectures, workshops, presentations and an after-school program. The newest program is an after-school dance program "Ballroom Social, Cultural dance program" working with underserved middle school children, ages eleven through fifteen. Partnerships provide important support, such as marketing services by the Hallandale Beach Chamber of Commerce, in order for the program to focus on the families of Gulf Stream Middle school children. ArtServe has worked with leadership to design and implement outreach to schools, youth and professionals.

Choreology Basic

The Hallandale Section of CID-UNESCO INC. has an MOU signed with the non-profit organization Multicultural Educational Center located in Miami-Dade. (funded by the Miami-Dade Department of Cultural Affairs) and the need to partner with non-profit organization USA Dance. These collaborations bridge the age divide between the younger members of the Dance community and the seasoned amateurs and professionals who dance, perform, and compete in the various venues and organizations. This past year, the team created a tv program through the school system and they are excited that in addition the local tv station will air their programs this year.

Hallandale has also piloted a medical program in a physician's office and are seeing healing through movement in many situations. Leaders would like to further this pilot program, so documentation and evaluative assessment should be in place to move the program forward.

Participants report that they are building the momentum one community as a time. They have worked with the Haitian community, and now are working with a Chinese community. They have successfully engaged with four counties including Boynton, Dade, Broward and Palm Beach and have Davie and Miami Counties coming aboard soon.

Future Needs: Fundraising and grant writing training will be key to high growth Determine how to engage people to be a part of the organizational programs Document the excitement and the impact on students to share with other school districts Institutionalize presentation packages to key government officials, board of education, so that board and volunteers will be able to participate in recruitment of partners and sponsorships.

MANAGEMENT & STAFFING Michel Francois Jacques is the founder and president of HSCID and serves as the volunteer artistic and administrative director. Mr. Jacques provides pro-bono office space now, as well as studio space in previous years. Mr. Jacques has attended the local grant writing workshop and has sought out grant writing assistance and is recruiting more active CID members. He understands that an organization is only as strong as its' committed members. The building of organizational capacity has been a challenge due to lack of funding. However, with the grant award from the Broward Cultural Division, they are confident in their ability to attract more funding.

The recruitment of volunteers is done on an ongoing basis and considered successful as evidenced by the in-kind hours of 3497 reported in 2016. Volunteers are trained on the use of effective techniques to deliver excellent customer service and fun recruiting techniques for the Annual Dance Congress. The training sessions are held in small groups and on an individual basis.

HALLANDALE SECTION CID 12/18 PAMELA KINGFISHER, SHINING WATERS CONSULTING

3
SUMMARY OF THE FACILITATED SELF-ASSESSMENT

MISSION AND HISTORY Hallandale Section of CID/UNESCO was incorporated in 2013 from the vision of Michel Jacques. After Michel went to a CID/UNESCO event and saw a new way to improve quality dance in America and to share with global audiences, he returned to Florida and founded the organization. This is the first UNESCO Dance (CID) in the US and their goal is to form a chapter in every city, county and state in the US.

Founded as a Florida nonprofit, the chapter has 25 active dance entrepreneurs as teachers who provide their expertise to schools, organizations, and businesses in order to improve quality dance in America to share with global audiences. Dance is an educational process, so Michele is bringing ballroom and cultural dances to the world as the President of US Section CID/INESCO. The vision of the organization is to fashion a safe and tolerant multicultural space where children of all ages can learn to express themselves.

The International Dance Council (CID) is the official umbrella organization for all forms of dance in all countries of the world and is recognized by UNESCO, national and local governments, international organizations and institutions. CID brings together the most important international, national and local organizations, as well as select individuals active in Dance.

Choreology Basic

Hallandale's' Section mission is: The mission of the Hallandale Section of CID-UNESCO INC. is to organize once a year the International Congress on Dance research studies. This program brings together dancers from different countries to participate, learn & experience the American cultural music & dance forms.

The goal of the CID USA Section is to serve the national UNESCO mission on a grassroots level, as an umbrella organization and a motivation for ballroom dance activities in the community, colleges, and schools. The organization is known for its' annual CID Dance Congress held in Broward County, Florida.

Much of the CID resources are devoted to promoting, organizing and supporting couples-dancing programs for youth and collegiate dancers at the collegiate and K-12 levels throughout the nation and fostering and helping sustain purposeful CID Sections throughout the United States. Providing youth with opportunities to "learn mutual trust and build respect between boys and girls and people of all ethnicities". This is not party dancing or freestyle, it is the art of dance and you can feel the difference. This is a way to exchange our cultures and have fun while making connections with others.

The broader goals of the CID partnership include encouragement of the Olympics Dance Sport category and a K-12 after school dance teachers' programs, support of seniors as recreational dancers, and fostering a healthy, productive cultural exchange through the general media, the CID USA website as well as social media sites and the CID-worldwide portal.

MARKET/AUDIENCE/PROGRAMS Program activities began with the introduction of the CID/UNESCO Dance Congress to South Florida. The Dance Congress includes a full program including research reports, lectures on original subjects such as dance history, and the physical and psychological effects of dance therapy. Workshops demonstrate various dance methods and skills, along with performances by dance companies, video projections and exhibitions and sales of books, records, pictures, and costumes.

Michel F. Jacques

HALLANDALE SECTION CID 12/18 PAMELA KINGFISHER, SHINING WATERS CONSULTING

2 Background Broward Cultural Division, the local arts agency for Broward County, commissioned this facilitated assessment for its Cultural Diversity Program grantee, Hallandale Section of CID/UNESCO. This assessment identifies key organizational development issues facing the organization that may provide the basis for its next four years of grant funding from Broward Cultural Division and subsequent opportunities for technical assistance. The Broward Cultural Division commissioned Shining Waters Consulting (through the local ArtServe organization) to facilitate organizational self-assessments in order to strengthen the organizational infrastructure and financial capacity of artist-centered organizations through group technical assistance.

The Self-Assessment Facilitation Process In advance of the assessment, the consultant reviewed available organizational materials. On site, the consultant facilitated assessment discussions with key representatives from the organization's staff, board, artists, and volunteers via a series of specific questions on the following topics:

1. The organization's mission and history, current market, audiences, and programming;

2. The current capacity and future requirements for its management and staffing, board of directors, and facilities;

3. The organization's recent financial performance as well as projected future financial needs; and

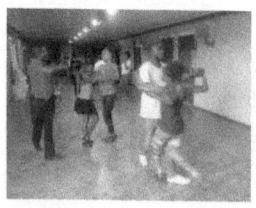
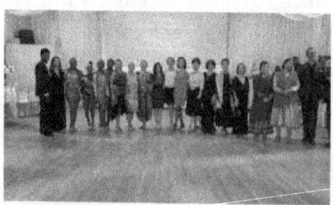

Choreology Basic

4. The adequacy of current administrative systems, marketing, and technology related to present and future needs.

At each stage of development, an organization can expect a variety of resource and structural incongruities that can distract it from complete fulfillment of its mission. These infrastructure issues present predictable challenges that require discretely different strategies at each stage.

Self-assessment participants identified the lifecycle stage for their organization as a whole, as well as for its programs, management, and board of directors, financial resources, and systems. We could thus note any components out of synch with others, as well as assess whether proposed uses of Initiative funds were appropriate given the organization's developmental stage. (Because the model was described to participants during their self-assessment, this report does not contain further explanation of its discrete phases; for additional information, please refer to Stevens' Nonprofit Lifecycles: Stage-based Wisdom for Nonprofit Capacity, 2002.)

We concluded the self-assessment by summarizing the critical issues identified throughout the day. Participants discussed how funding resources (grants and technical assistance) could be most strategically applied in light of self-assessment findings.

List of self-assessment participants: President: Mr. Michel F Jacques Vice-President: Ms. Lori-Nan Kaye Treasurer: Marie Margaret Charles Hallandale Section of CID/UNESCO.

Self-Assessment of Organizational Capacity

December 2018

Prepared by: Pamela Kingfisher, Principal Shining Waters Consulting

New Board of Management: Michel F. Jacques President/Founder Olga Miele Katz first Vice President, Dr. Cheryl White Seconde Vice President, Rita Singer Treasurer, Stanley Jacques Ex. Secretary

Michel F. Jacques

My question is: What are we listening to when dancing? What are we listening to when walking on the Beach or exercising on a treadmill etc. Are you dancing or thinking?

I have been observing a decline of civilization in the entertainment industry. Dancers sometimes confuse internal rhythm with rhythm within music. The confusion is between the intra-personnel dialogue and the inter-personnel communication. A make belief tactic in the dance art forms affects our youth health and wellness. We tend to dance for fun or just for individual interest, Leads our youth to the streets with lack of discipline & etiquettes.

The fact is when it comes to Dance, we all need to listen to music rhythm the right way. Rhythm as sacred & a spiritual element within music cannot be changed. Dancing is a form of prayer, a dialogue with the architect of the Universe guides us to live an everlasting life. All rhythms came from the Cosmos and the Divine. In the mind of a choreographer death should not exist.

Dancing off timing to music is considered a misinterpretation of rhythm, leading our dancers to develop lack of concentration, and respect to the artist musician who creates it.

Children dance practitioners tend to develop multiple chronic feeling disorders, stresses, lack of concentration and respect between themselves. Apparently they are confused and would not understand and follow laws that governs nature, nations Etc.

Dancing is the equivalence of music. Why there are Universities all over the world where young adult can go for a career in music. There are not enough school yet for dance educators. The reason why this book is written as a remedy for change toward a better dancing community.

How old is the earth? Is the Earth 4.5 billion years old or only 6000 years old as the Bible teaches? Evolutionists fallaciously think that

Choreology Basic

billions of years of time makes particles-to-people evolution possible. According to experts, the Bible states that man was made six days after creation, about 6,000 years ago. The Bible says the earth is about 6000 years old. Evolution says the earth is billions of years old. What is the truth? Good News Tube is a channel of Christian videos sharing the good news of God's Kingdom. Are you feeling unloved, lonely, depressed, and anxious, like there's no purpose for your life and no hope for your future? The good news is that God loves you, he has a wonderful plan for your life and a glorious future for you in Heaven with him. Good News Tube wants to share the good news of the gospel with you by way of Christian videos and playlists with a positive uplifting message from Jesus. By subscribing to Good News Tube you will learn more about the Christian faith from the world's best evangelists like Doug Batchelor, David Asscherick, John Bradshaw, Stephen Bohr. You will find the answers to some of life's tough questions. You will also learn about creation and Bible prophecy. Best of all you will find peace, happiness and eternal life through Jesus Christ. Subscribe now!

"Evolution says the earth is billions of years old". One said, No. Evolution is simply the process of life on earth. Physics, Geology, Chemistry, Astronomy, Paleontology, Archeology, etc. have all shown the earth is 4.5 billion years old based upon EVIDENCE.

This fast-moving video probes the reaches of space, revealing the awesome power of our Creator. Featuring the acclaimed Creation Museum planetarium program designed by astrophysicist Jason Lisle, it reveals amazing facts about our universe while exalting God as creator.

Using state-of-the-art animation, viewers are taken on a journey beyond our solar system to the edge of the known universe. Created Cosmos, will take you thousands of light-years between billions of planets, stars, nebulae, and galaxies to discover the magnitude of our universe and of its Creator. GoodNews Tube is a channel of Christian videos sharing the good news of God's Kingdom.

Are you feeling unloved, lonely, depressed, and anxious, like there's no purpose for your life and no hope for your future? The good news is that God loves you, he has a wonderful plan for your life and a glorious future for you in Heaven with him. Good News Tube wants to share the good news of the gospel with you by way of Christian videos and playlists with a positive uplifting message from Jesus. By subscribing to Good News Tube you will learn more about the Christian faith from the world's best evangelists like Doug Batchelor, David Asscherick, John Bradshaw, Stephen Bohr.

You will find the answers to some of life's toughest questions. You will also learn about creation and Bible prophecy. Best of all you will find peace, happiness and eternal life and healing through dance.

DANCING AS A TOOL OF CULTURAL DIPLOMACY

Research By: Marcela Zia[1]

1. INTRODUCTION

In the current increasingly globalized world, individuals, corporations and governments from across the globe are becoming more integrated than ever before and have the ability to exchange information faster and more efficiently. Considering that there is a growing interdependency between nations, the development of lasting bilateral relations and based on mutual trust would be required. In this sense, international relations must be seen not only through the prism of political and economic understanding, but also from the cultural aspect, since culture can facilitate the process of regional and global integration. Thus, inter-cultural relations have become increasingly important in the 21st century, as they lead to a better understanding and greater trust between cultures, prevent

---

[1] Member of the International Dance Council – CID UNESCO and Student of the Masters Program in Dance at the Institute of Arts of the State University of Campinas, Brazil (UNICAMP).

misunderstanding, improve communication and cooperation and help to reduce the likelihood of socio-cultural conflicts.

In today's turbulent political world, diplomacy means play a crucial role in a country's efforts to achieve political goals and to promote its image in the international arena. No democratic country relies solely on military and economic means in its interactions with other countries. Rather, all maintain Ministries of Foreign Affairs whose goal is to interact with other countries via diplomatic channels.

Cultural diplomacy is the use of cultural activities as an additional element of enabling partnerships, that means, culture is used as a tool for bringing countries together. Through international projection of its values, the country will have chances to build a positive image abroad which may result in achieving greater international prestige. Cultural diplomacy has long been recognized as a prime instrument to promote international links and understanding between countries and peoples.

The objective of this paper is to establish what are the aims and the benefits of cultural diplomacy and to analyze how dance can be used as a toll of cultural diplomacy. In order to illustrate how dance can be important and relevant to integrate people and countries and to build a country's image abroad, we will focus on two outstanding programs of cultural diplomacy developed by the governments of the United States and Soviet Union during the Cold War. Both countries were investing in exporting their dancers abroad in order to show their ideologies and to project a positive image in the international arena.

2. CULTURAL DIPLOMACY: DEFINITION AND IMPORTANCE

2.1 – Definition of Cultural diplomacy

According to Dr. Emil Constantinescu, President of the Academy for Cultural Diplomacy, Cultural Diplomacy may be best described as a course of actions, which are based on and utilize the exchange of ideas, values, traditions and other aspects of culture or identity, whether to strengthen relationships, enhance socio-cultural cooperation or promote national interests; Cultural diplomacy can be practiced by either the public sector, private sector or civil society.[2]

Although there is no set or commonly agreed upon definition of cultural diplomacy, it can be defined as the means through which countries promote their cultural and political values to the rest of the world. The essential idea is to allow people access to different cultures and perspectives, and in this way, foster mutual understanding and dialogue.

Culture is an exceedingly broad term, thus contributing to the vast range of areas that fall under the definition of cultural diplomacy. Edgar Telles Ribeiro, based on anthropological concepts, defines culture as "... the sum of habits, customs and achievements of an individual, a community, a people over its history." Further, " ... these achievements embraces all fields of human activity, from the arts to science, from technology to folklore, from politics to religion, from health to sport, from trade to leisure.[3] In short, everything would be culture. In these ways, culture includes literature, the arts in general, customs, habits and traditions, human's behavior, history, dance, music, folklore, gestures and social relationships. Thus, any interaction or exchange between people of two countries in any of these areas can be considered cultural diplomacy.

2.2 – The importance of Cultural diplomacy

≫ For the preservation of Global Peace & Stability

In an increasingly globalized, interdependent world, in which the proliferation of mass communication technology ensures we all have greater access to each other than ever before, cultural diplomacy is critical

---

[2] Institut for Cultural Diplomacy. (2015, September 08) Retrieved from www.culturaldiplomacy.org
[3] RIBEIRO, EDGAR TELLES. **Diplomacia Cultural – Seu papel na Política Externa Brasileira**. Brasília: Fundação Alexandre Gusmão, 1989, p. 19.

to fostering peace and stability throughout the world. Cultural diplomacy, when learned and applied at all levels, possesses the unique ability to influence the "Global Public Opinion" and ideology of individuals, communities, culture or nations. The exchange of experiences, ideas and valuable assets of a nation to another, allows the establishment of an atmosphere favorable for understanding. Therefore, even if the cultural events are modest, they always reinforce a certain degree of communion, contributing to the rapprochement of peoples and cultures.

The Institute for Cultural Diplomacy describes 5 principles that can be accomplished with the use of cultural diplomacy. The realization of the first principle enables the second, which in turn enables the third until the fifth ultimate principle of global peace and stability is achieved.

The principles are:

1- Respect and Recognition of Cultural Diversity & Heritage;
2- Global Intercultural Dialogue;
3- Justice, Equality & Interdependence;
4- The Protection of International Human Rights; 5- Global Peace & Stability. [4]

▶▶ For political relations

Cultural diplomacy is in essence the mobilization of what the political scientist Prof. Joseph Nye referred to as "soft power". Nye stipulates that "the soft power of a country rests primarily on three sources; its culture…, its political values.. and its foreign policies.". He has made a distinction between two approaches that are used to conduct regional and international relations: hard power and soft power: "The ability to persuade through culture, values and ideas, as opposed to "hard power", which conquers or coerces thorough military might". [5] Whilst the 'hard

---

[4] Institut for Cultural Diplomacy. (2015, September 08) Retrieved from www.culturaldiplomacy.org
[5] NYE, JOSEPH (2004). **Soft Power: The Means to Success in World Politics,** 5. Public Affairs, New York.

power' approach has historically been a favored policy of governments in conducting international and regional relations, the increasingly interconnected world stage highlights the need for co-operation on a new level. This is where the role of Soft Power as a form of cultural diplomacy becomes significant. On this basis, cultural diplomacy is not secondary to political or economic diplomacy, but rather functions as an intrinsic and necessary component of it.

The author RIBEIRO says that cultural relations have the ability to raise awareness beyond political or economic limits, after all, "the military or economic power of a nation tends to intimidate, while culture tends to seduce."[6]

▶▶ For International Business

As the move towards more socially responsible business practices gains momentum, the ability to understand and embrace the different values and needs of diverse cultures and societies becomes ever more important. There are many reasons why corporations need to be aware of the differences between cultures in their strategic decision-making process and adopt cultural diplomacy models into their agenda:

- In the era of growing social awareness, corporates with culturally sensitive marketing plans and campaigns will enjoy a positive public opinion and good image, thus financially perform better.

- Companies seeking to expand abroad, will encounter problems unless they conduct research into, and act according to the cultural differences with the host country.

- Companies with a national focus face a related challenge in ensuring that they are aware of and sensitive to national cultural minorities.

---

[6] RIBEIRO, EDGAR TELLES. **Op. Cit.** p. 26

Additionally, cultural activities encourage the strengthening of a climate of confidence in commercial relations and in the qualifications of the countries. By demonstrating their ability in culture, the country will also be drawing attention implicitly to their qualifications in other areas.[7]

➢➢ In the field of Education

One of the most important fields in which cultural diplomacy can reap important benefits is the field of education. Around the world, cultural diplomacy has penetrated the field of education in the past and continues to do so today. Textbooks in secondary school and universities are often inundated with information about the cultures of different countries, religions, and ethnic groups. Such efforts are often designed to educate children to understand and respect the traditions and lifestyles of people of other nationalities. Many universities around the world offer students the opportunity to spend a semester abroad, immersing themselves in the culture of a foreign country.

➢➢ In the field of Arts

An additional field which has witnessed an inundation of cultural diplomacy programs around the world over the past few years is the sphere of arts. As part of cultural diplomacy programs, countries may send artists abroad to display their exhibits in foreign countries or may host foreign artists at international exhibitions on their own soil. Such interactions enhance knowledge and correct stereotypes, preparing the ground for a more open environment for diplomatic and political relations. Through international arts exchanges a country can demonstrate to other countries around the world just how developed and sophisticated it is in the field of arts and can succeed in dispelling various negative stereotypes that people in other countries may harbor toward it.

---

[7] **Id. Ibid**. P. 28-30

Michel F. Jacques

3. DANCE AS A TOOL OF CULTURAL DIPLOMACY

Since a long time dance is used as a tool of cultural diplomacy. Throughout history, there are numerous programs developed by countries around the world that focused on exporting dance artists abroad in order to export, simultaneously, a certain image or ideology of the nation. This paper will focus on the early decades of the Cold War, periods when United States and Soviet Union sent artists, as well as art objects, abroad as part of its cultural diplomacy programs. This cultural competition between two major powers proved unprecedented as each side sought to use every instance of cultural exchange to attract support and to demonstrate its system's superiority.

On one hand, as an example of a Soviet cultural diplomatic effort, we have the Bolshoi Ballet's American Premiere, That occurred in 1959. Soviet officials resolved to utilize the Bolshoi Ballet's planned 1959 American tour to awe audiences with Soviet choreographers' great accomplishments and Soviet performers' superb abilities. The repertoire included the four ballets, Romeo and Juliet, Swan Lake, Giselle, and The Stone Flower, and two Highlights Programs, which included excerpts from various pre- and post-revolutionary ballets, operas, and dance suites. How the Americans and the Soviets understood the Bolshoi's success provides insight into how each side conceptualized the role of the arts in society and in political transformation.

When the Soviet leadership determined to use cultural diplomacy, as a weapon in the Cold War, they believed that this plan would prove effective in exporting Communism's achievements and for attracting American supporters. The Soviet leadership concluded that applause for the Bolshoi was really applause for the Soviet system, and could therefore conclude that the Bolshoi's performances were lessening Americans' anti-Communist sentiments. This weakening of Americans' anti-Soviet

For instance was an important Cold War victory that would eventually lead to the Soviet Union's ultimate victory over capitalism.[8]

On the other hand, the U.S. President Dwight D. Eisenhower launched the exchange program that sent American dancers and choreographers to countries with which he had political relations. The idea was to use dance to export an idealized image of America and also to combat Soviet influence around the world, thus diminishing the spread of communism. In order to disseminate the American culture and to demonstrate their ideals of freedom through a more innovative and modern dance, the government encouraged the organization of international tours of several dance companies, such as: José Limón to South America, Martha Graham to Asia, Alvin Ailey to the South Pacific and George Balanchine to Western Europe, Japan and the Soviet Union.[9] The goal was to influence hearts and minds in other countries, and to show that military might and commercial interests were not the only things Americans valued.[10]

It was true in the Cold Was period and it is true today, that the power of the dance as a toll of cultural diplomacy may not be quantifiable, but have enormous contribution on the foreign policy of the countries, once it allows building a certain image of the nation, exporting a ideology, and also promotes a peaceful environment.

BIBLIOGRAFY

1. RIBEIRO, Edgard Telles. **Diplomacia Cultural: Seu papel na Política Externa Brasileira.** Brasília: Fundação Alexandre

---

[8] MCDANIEL, CADRA PETERSON. **Soviet Cultural Diplomacy – The Bolshoi Ballet's American Premiere**. Lexington Books, 1984.
[9] PREVOTS, NAIMA. **Dance for Export – Cultural Diplomacy and the Cold War**. Wesleyan University Press, 1998.
[10] PREVOTS, NAIMA. **Dance and the Cold War – Exports to Latin America**. (September, 08th, 2015).
Revista Harvard Review of Latin America. Harvart University. Retrieved from: http://revista.drclas.harvard.edu/book/dance-and-cold-war

Gusmão / Instituto de Pesquisa de Relações Internacionais, 1989, 102 p.

2. Institut for Cultural Diplomacy. (2015, September 08) Retrieved from www.culturaldiplomacy.org

3. NYE, JOSEPH (2004). **Soft Power: The Means to Success in World Politics,** 5. Public Affairs, New York.

4. MCDANIEL, CADRA PETERSON. **Soviet Cultural Diplomacy – The Bolshoi Ballet's American Premiere**. Lexington Books, 1984.

5. PREVOTS, NAIMA. **Dance for Export – Cultural Diplomacy and the Cold War.** Wesleyan University Press, 1998.

6. PREVOTS, NAIMA. **Dance and the Cold War – Exports to Latin America**. (September, 08th, 2015). Revista Harvard Review of Latin America. Harvart University. retrieved from: http://revista.drclas.harvard.edu/book/dance-and-cold-war

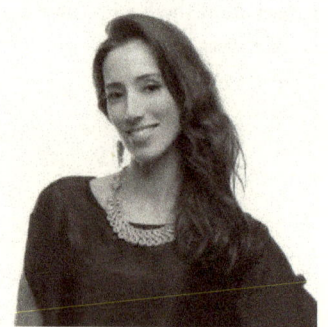

Marcela Zia

70 YEARS OF BALLET ART IN THE REPUBLIC OF NORTH MACEDONIA

Abstract

The proposed presentation gives an overview of the seventy year period of ballet art existence in the Republic of North Macedonia. The author had divided the relatively long period of time into four periods, conditionally. Basically, the research analyzes and systematizes settled repertoire ballet works. Within the framework of the National Theater, besides conducting drama and opera performances, in the year of 1949, for the very first time on its stage, the ballet art appears as a new theatrical genre. The first period is a period of enthusiasm and staffing along a huge repertoire challenges facing the classical ballet. The second period represents the affirmation of artistic demands facing contemporary ballet trends in Europe. The third period is characterized by creative processes that strengthen their own paths of ballet development. The fourth and nowadays period, represents the challenge towards globalization and integration in the art field as well as fostering national dance expression.

Keywords

Ballet art, historical approaches in North Macedonia, tradition, contemporaneity

Michel F. Jacques

Introduction

First period

The emergence of ballet art in North Macedonia - New theatrical genre within the Macedonian National Theater

The numerous musical and dance achievements of European folk cultures represent the very foundation whereof the ballet art rises as a highest form of stage dance art. Risen up in the Renaissance era courts performances, it finds its own way to the Balkans many centuries later.

After the Second World War, in 1945, the first independent national theater was created, which began the process of adopting the best achievements in the field of ballet art. During the first few years, only the Drama department performed on National Theater's stage, then in 1948 the Opera joined the Drama Theater, as in 1948/49 the image of National Theatre was enriched with the third branch of stage art – the ballet art. The immensely rich national folklore and folks innate dance ability are counted as factors that allow inspiration, retrospective acceptance of foreign historical experience and the birth of a new dance quality – the ballet art in North Macedonia.

The historical moment of the birth of a national ballet art relates to the name of Macedonian ballet founder - George Macedonian. As a chief of the Ballet at Skopje State Opera, he was

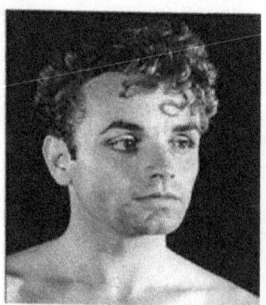

George Macedonian
ballet founder in North Macedonia

Choreology Basic

Appointed on July 1, 1948, as he onetime says in an interview, is appointed for the Head of the Ballet – "The Ballet that did not yet existed". The desire to adopt the European classical dance system is even greater than the basic prerequisite for the emergence of ballet art in any Theater, as that is the existence of an educational institution for ballet staff teaching. It is the first distinguished specific of creating the Macedonian ballet.

The guidelines for ballet art future development are carefully plotted in the direction of overcoming the traditional knowledge. January 27, 1949 represents a bright date in the ballet history, noted with the premiere of the "Walpurgic Night" ballet by Charles Guno's "Faust" Opera, performed by a newly formed ballet collective.The season`s culmination is marked with the all-night ballet "Bahchissar Fountain" by Boris Asafiev, premiered on December 30, 1949.

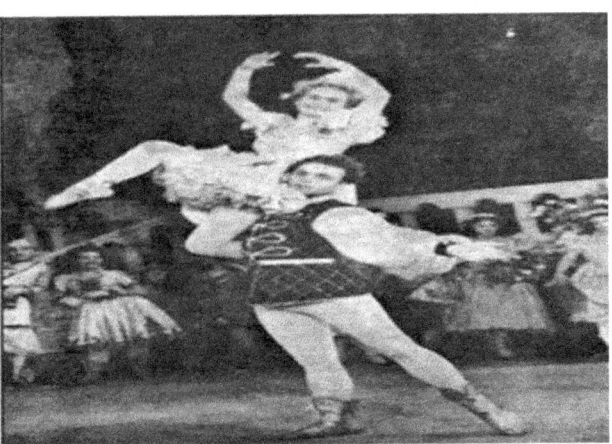

Penushliska and G.Macedonian
in Bahchissar Fountain, year of 1949

The phase of adolescence follows a firmly established guidelines of mastering the classical system as universal, accessible to every culture and nation. This period of enormous enthusiasm and love towards dancing is unseen in this region which characterizes the overall cultural rise of the young Macedonian Republic.

Michel F. Jacques

In the National Theater, the educational process goes hand in hand with the process of implementing performances with rich classical heritage. The choice of performances is specific and speaks to the following.

At the beginning of the 20th century the influence of Diagillev's "Paris Seasons" into the West was enormous. The richness of Russian classical school has been revealed through them as they are the herald of domination in the Russian ballet throughout the 20th century.This is due to the fact that national schools and theaters were formed in Europe under the influence of the "Russian seasons". This process has an impact in North Macedonia as well, since the first ballet dancers in the North Macedonian National Theater, as George Macedonain, Aleksandar Dobrohov, Nina Kirsanova, Dimitrie Parlic, are directly linked to the Russian classical school.

The stage performances, during the early period, had been a part of Diagilev's ballet repertoire.

The method of educating the ballet staff, the selection of the first pedagogues-choreographers repertoire, confirms the fact of close connection with everything that happens in the ballet theater in borders of then so called country - Yugoslavia as well as in Europe. From this point on, the roots of the ballet art in North Macedonia has been clearly illuminated.

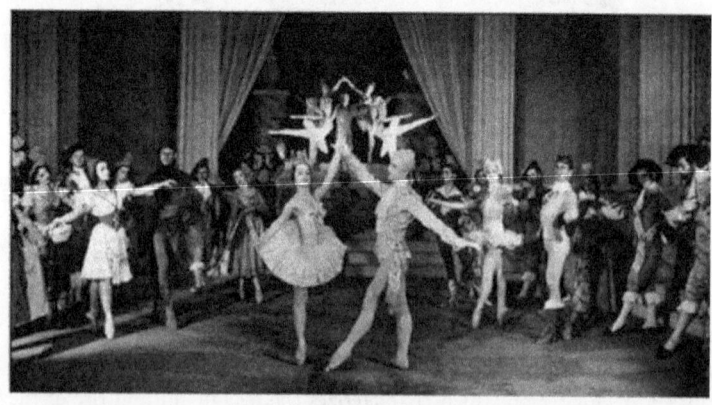

„Sleeping beauty", by choreographer N.Kirsanova, year of 1955

Choreology Basic

Whats most appealing, is that, during the adoption of ballet art in a short period of time, the theater activists strove towards an ancient North Macedonian folklore tradition ballet implementation. The Composer Gligor Smokvarski composes the music for the first national ballet "Macedonian Entry" (1953), performed in choreography by renowned Yugoslavian choreographer Dimitrie Parlic.

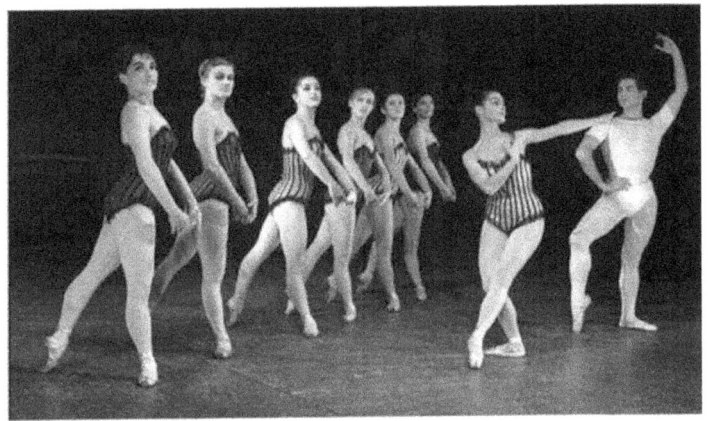

„Impression", choreographer D.Parlic, year of 1953

The initial period of creating the ballet art in today's Republic of North Macedonia can be summarized in a timeframe of 1948-1965, conditionally.

The entire professional activity in this period rests on the work of the above-mentioned pedagogues and choreographers who set out the classical heritage ballets: "Second Rhapsody" -1952; "Polovetsky Camp"-1952; "On the Ball"-1953; "Scheherazade"-1953; "Coppelia" -1954; "Sleeping Beauty"-1955; "Giselle"-1956; "Swan Lake"-1957; "Sulfides"-1957; "Wizard's Love" -1962; "Romeo and Juliet" -1962.

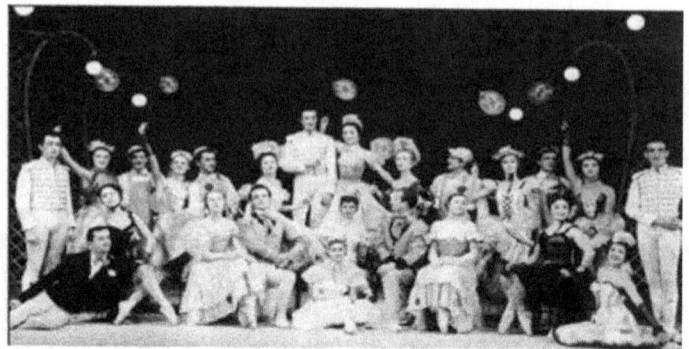

"Straussiade", by choreographer N.Kirsanova, year of 1956 – after premier

From the ballet creation policy's point of view which had not existed in this region a time before, the already set ballets were seen as a professional choice with exceptional importance.

Through their pedagogical work and set stage achievements in National Theatre, we find the outlines of the parallels that move the Macedonian ballet, as well as its intertwining with the artistic achievements in Yugoslavia and its closeness to the latest aesthetic demands of ballet art in Europe. This speaks for a high professionalism and comprehensive cultural cooperation. The set works by the founders of the Macedonian Ballet make this fact undeniable.

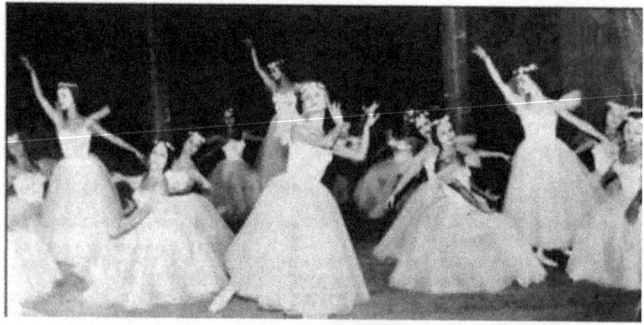

"Sulfides", in choreography by N.Kirsanova, year of 1957

Choreology Basic

Second period

Period of challenges-Affirmation of artistic exploration facing contemporary ballet trends

The next period of the Macedonian National Theater ballet art development is connected to the opening of mount theater installation. After the old building was demolished in the catastrophic 1963 earthquake in Skopje, mount theater installation became the second temporary home scene on which the ballet collective operated.

The second period is characterized by the affirmation of creative research, focused towards the contemporary world trends. Orderly, the new challenges were rooted in the previous period. That is why the artistic period of the second time chapter has to be seen in a conditional time frame from 1965 to 1983.

In this context, we refer to the visit of Jose Lemon's American troops to Skopje in 1957. In Lemon's choreographies, the elaborations of social and ethical-philosophical themes have a strong emotional charge in the viewer. The very visit has an influence over exposing the enormous contemporary expressive possibilities of the ballet. It takes just one spark of domestic ballet figures to inflame the desires for a new art of dance repertoire conquests.

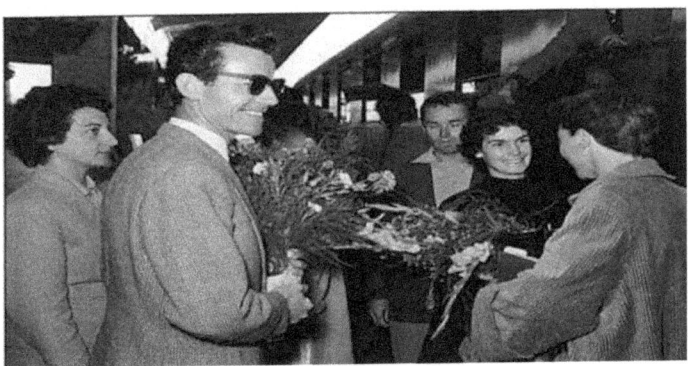

Michel F. Jacques

> Jovan Pashti, Natka Penushliska, Georg Macedonian welcome the members of the American Ballet troupe at the Skopje Railway Station

After the retrospective adoption of the classics in the initial first period of ballet art development, in the second period, the challenges are directed towards new demands in theater politics. The repertoire conceptualization represents the most complex problem to be solved in the Theaters, as the Macedonian National Theater. A dedication towards presenting performances with a contemporary ballet express, represents a valuable diversity in enriching the repertoire. Starting from the total number, out of 42 performances played in this period, more than half are contemporary, or 22 in number. Adding to this figure are the musical performances by the home composers, which also have a contemporary choreographic expression, and by which we come to the upper hand of repertoire of contemporary ballets over the classical ones.

The attitude of the Theater Directorate towards national music creation and the introduction of modern-oriented works is a far-reaching caring step in the repertoire policy, a step that will continue in the future time period.

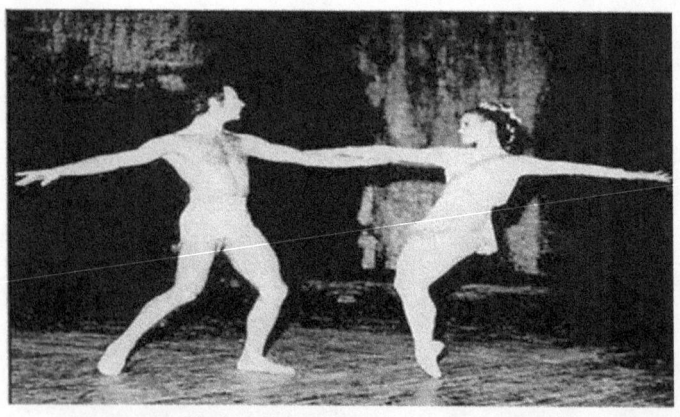

N.Penushliska, M.Crvenov in „Song over songs", in choreography by Fragno Chorvat, year of 1967

Choreology Basic

Addressing the domestic musical creation is seen as a basic feature that characterizes this period of national ballet art development. Taken from its side, it draws a plethora of choreographers from the ranks of Macedonian ballet artists as: Olga Milosavlova, Marin Crvenov, Aleksandar Stojanovic, Ekrem Hussein. In the exceptionally rich repertoire register of home-made works, we note the names of the following home composers: Trajko Prokopiev with the ballet "Labin and Dojrana"; Toma Proshev - "Frames and Echoes", "Song over Songs", "Waves", "Poem"; the composer Ljubomir Brangolica with the ballets "Metropolis Variations", "Abolition", "Blind Girl", "Military Story", "Reflection", "It's a Man", "Kara Mita"; then the composer Tomislav Zografski - "Journeys"; Blagoja Ivanovski - "Frescoes"; Aleksandar Lekovski – "Aspirations".

The source of the national juices on which the mix of domestic music-choreographic requirements has been set is remarkably rich. The repertoire is enriched with colorful freshness and recognition. The Macedonian creators (composers, choreographers) draw the inexhaustible power of artistic inspiration from its roots, continuing the tradition. From a historical point of view, it is a process of a deep need and resilient endurance in the continuity of one's own existence.

At the crossroad of choosing the path for their future development, the national theater was solving the problems along the way. The young ballet staff lacks their own educated staff considering profiles like ballet pedagogues, repeaters, choreographers. This is complemented by inviting guests from abroad. The strong determination of the ballet troupe at the National Theater to develop itself according to the laws of strong classical heritage repertoire continues in this period precisely through the work of foreign ballet experts.

During this period, the Russian professor Yuri Miyachin gave an unselfish help in order to resolve the repertoire policy of the already mature Macedonian ballet dancers, setting the ballets "Raymonda", "Don Quixote" "Ballet Concert" on the stage in Skopje, as he featured classical heritage pearls.

Michel F. Jacques

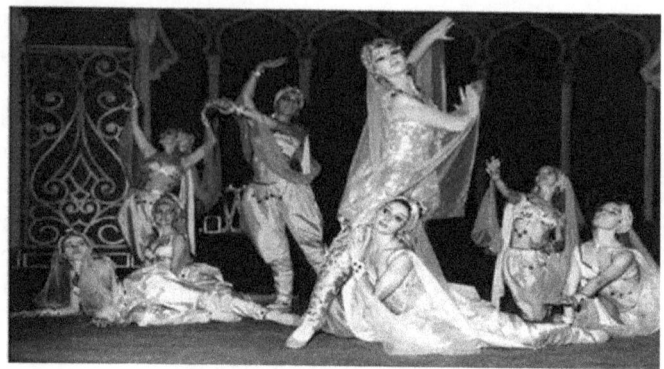

Vera Brangolica in „Ohrid legend"

The efforts given by many foreign guest pedagogues, choreographers are deeply embedded in the history of Macedonian ballet. That process of connection continues to live. In it lies the specificity and beauty of the ballet.

The conclusion that we can clearly draw out, points towards the link between the Macedonian ballet and all contemporary tendencies that we find in European ballet art. The international roots, embedded in the basis of the plastic expression of the human body in the ballet performance, are adopted and complemented by the plastic expression of the Macedonian ballet artists. That link between cultures, present in the repertoire of our stage, lifts ballet art on a par with other theatrical arts in our country.

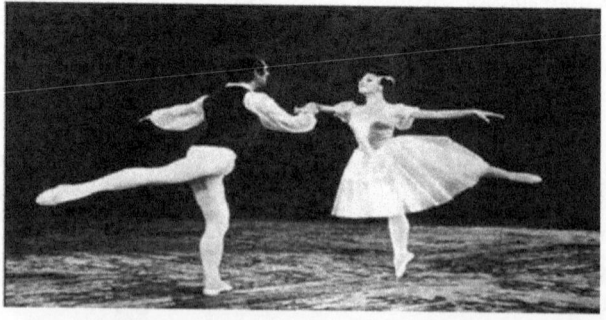

S.Spasevska Filipovska, M.Crvenov in „Giselle", year of 1978

Choreology Basic

Third period

Relevant creative processes – Unveiling and strengthening the own paths of development

The next period in the development of ballet art begins with the opening of a new theater building in the year of 1983. Conditionally, this period had completed within the year of 2004, when the Government of the Republic of Macedonia made a decision for establishing two national institutions. The old name - Macedonian National Theater (MNT) retains within the Drama, while the second national institution gets the name National Opera and Ballet.

After two decades of working in a mount theater installation, the opening of a new stage was spectacular, along the implementation of the ballet "Legend of Love" by composer A.Melikov. The stage, suitable for ballet performances, contributed towards a remarkably visual ballet art perception. A part of the credit for the performances's success, besides the soloists and ensemble, was given to a guest, the Ukrainian choreographer Anatoly Chikera.

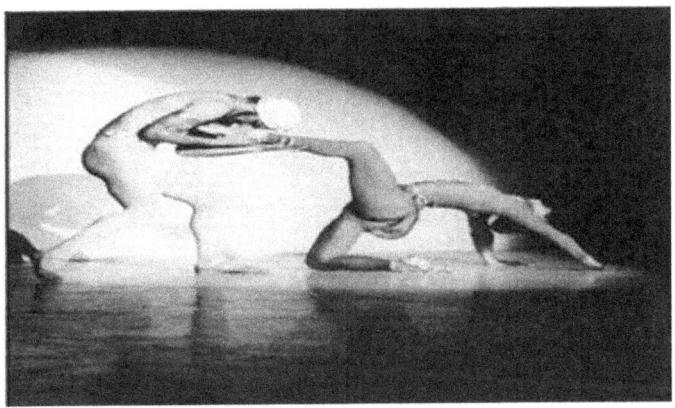

Zoica Purovska and Zoran Velevski in "Legend of Love", year of 1983

During the third period, the artistic developments' general features continues in the direction of strengthening their own paths. Given the wholesome on the achieved so far, the focus is on creative processes that are relevant to the advancement of ballet art.

As like in previous periods, misunderstandings, artistic disagreements, and insufficient care for staff and repertoire policies are also encountered in this period. Since 1979, Ballet has separated itself from the Opera and has acted as a stand-alone unit within the National Theater. Past problems are solved by the ballet staff and they were given a new flow. Analyzing the best performances in the repertoire, we also highlight the significant moments of the troupe's artistic growth and the individuals within it.

In the artistic sense of the word, the main driving force in the historical development of the national ballet troupe in the Republic of North Macedonia is two tendencies struggling for dominance. They periodically prevail over each other but also complement each other. The first tendency is to favor innovation, by expressing one's feelings and situations in which the human is placed in contemporary living conditions. Experimenting and searching for a new artistic expression does not always produce the desired productive results.

Fortunately, some of the performances in this period, such as the ballets "Carmina Burana", "Pink Floyd", "Pastels", "Zodiac" are a good opportunity to see the magnitude of the true domination of the artwork.

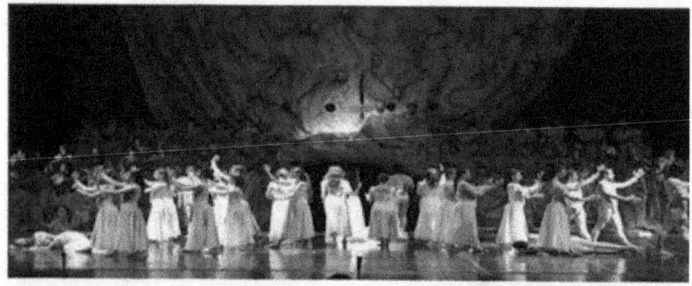

„Carmina Burana", with choreography by D. Boldin, year of 1991

Choreology Basic

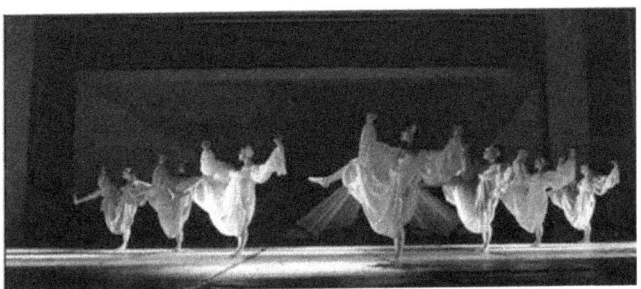

„Pink Floyd Revisited ", year of 1991

The second tendency that seeks towards the classical heritage ballets is a kind of equilibrium. Representation in the classical repertoire is the strongest basis for a proper conditional and technical progress of a national ballet troupe. In this period, the cooperation with foreign guests continues. It is worth mentioning the long-standing collaboration with people artist of Russia, Mikhail Krapivin, which results in passing on performances that are of a highest quality in our stage such as ballets: "Corsar", "Nutcracker", "Esmeralda", "Scheherazade". etc.

This rule of cyclical deviation, that is, the tendency to respect tradition or the greater prevalence of innovative ballet continues at length.

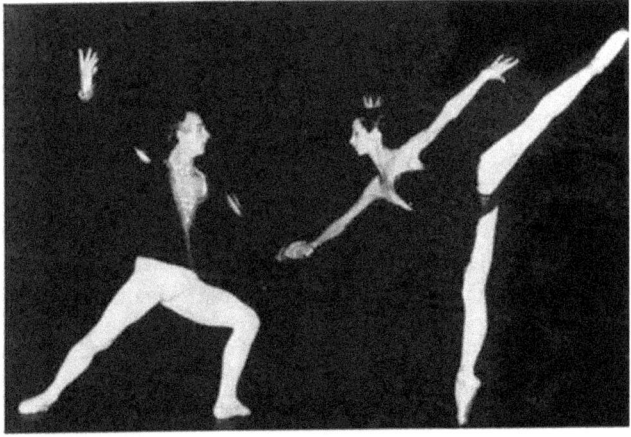

Tania Vuysich and Marin Crvenov in Swan Lake in the year 1986

Michel F. Jacques

In perpetuity setting performances, pre-performances of domestic composers, is also a very important part of the repertoire policy. The period we are talking about is particularly rich in domestic stage works and can be set aside as a basis on which the new generations future creative activity upgrades. Along her numerous choreographies, Olga Milosavlova is one of the most productive choreographers. The set of 14 ballets, in collaboration with the local composers, leave a strong mark in the specifical music-dance expression of the ballet actors on stage and as such has been an integral part of the unique Macedonian ballet tradition.

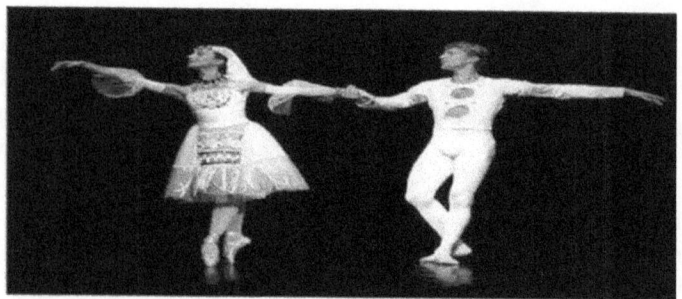

K.Kiprovska and C.Kostyukov in „Macedonian Entry", year of 1993

Following the conclusion, the historical achievements of the past fertilize the soil for future development of the modern ballet theater in North Macedonia. This process of national dance manifestation in its highest expressive art form – as ballet performance, is one of the most complex art processes. For years it chooses and puts its specific forms and means of expression, for years it elaborates them and through the modern dance-plastic language teaches new colors from the spectrum of human emotions. In this way the best artistic traditions, pass on to us from the world classical ballet heritage and complemented by the national sense of dance expression, are being preserved and modernized, thereby elevating ballet art to the level of high achievements in other arts (drama, opera, music creativity, etc.).

Choreology Basic

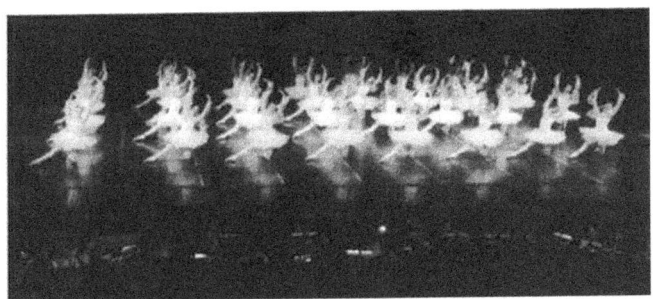

„La Bayadère", year of 1994

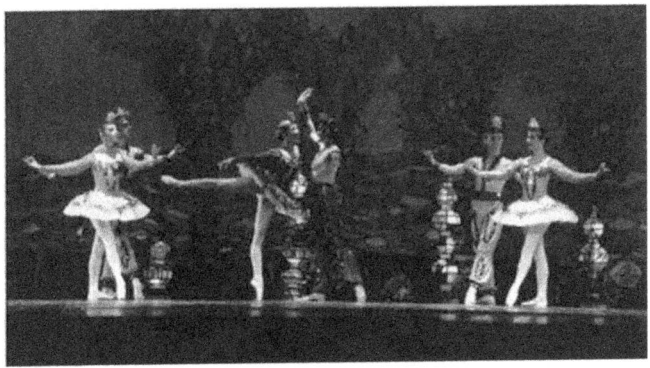

„Le Corsaire", year of 1996

Forth period

The national sense for expressing dance under the terms of world globalization and intergration – quintessence continuance of a created tradition

The ballet art developments' last period on the stage of National Institution of the Opera and Ballet, covers the period from the year 2004 until today. Analyzing the repertoire, as a mirror of development, we can conclude that the repertoire policy pursues the general characteristics of the so far artistic development. That being so, the presence of classical ballets in balance with the contemporary and national ballets continues. The last ones are increasingly reflecting the process of world globalization and cultural integration.

In context of this period, what we especially want to emphasize, is the fact that the created ballet tradition in North Macedonia, under the contemporary conditions of existence, retains the ability to preserve the mentality of the national dance culture, its independence and its qualitative determination. The national sense of dance expression can be felt in the best contemporary ballets which are set on our domestic stage.

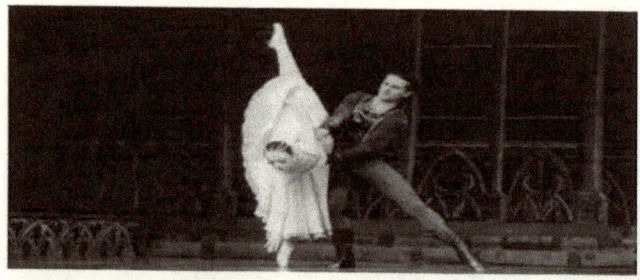

Natasha Nikolova, Vasiliy Chichiyashvilie in „Esmeralda", the year of 2005

The research shows that in the formatted ballet performances, the essence of the Macedonian dance genesis is visible through its incorporation into international ballet art. The very system of classical dance allows it as for that is open as a system. "The classic lives so that renewing itself, it does not disturb its foundations. It's always on the move and that's its strength. "(Федор Лопухов, „Хореографические откровенности", „Искусство", 1972 год, стр.24)

In its centuries-old existence the classical system absorbs the fresh juices of new dance appearances among the folks but at the same time allows the growth and recognition of national and cultural identity. This confirmed theatrical truth is build on the harmonious relationship between tradition and innovation in hereby ballet art.

Choreology Basic

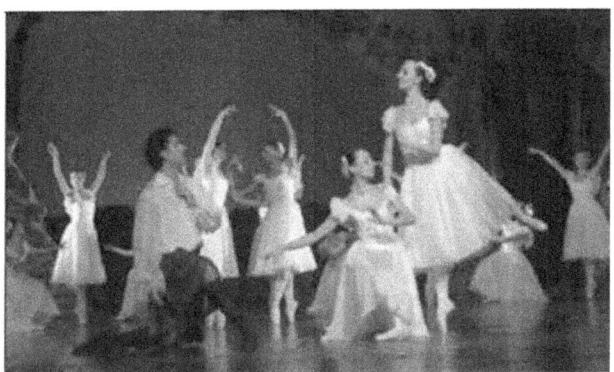

N.Nikolova, V.Chichiyashvilie, M. Yosifovska in „Les Sylphides"

The deviations process in ballet art development, with insufficient representation of all kinds of theater plays are harmful in a theatre house, such as our theater. Historically, alternate falls and ballet raises are seen as the result of several factors. One of the most important factors is the ignorance of the richness of the dance's expressive possibilities in contemporary aspiring performances. In that order, in the discussion, we would focus on dance as a leading component of synthetic ballet performance.

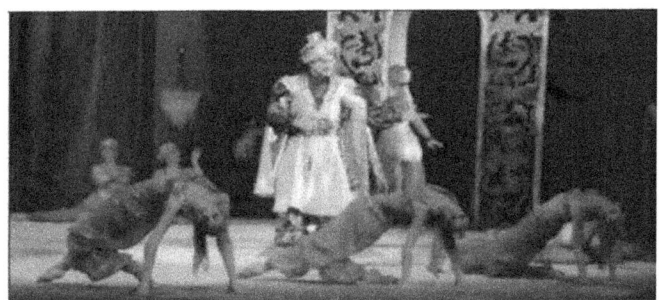

„Scheherazade", year of 2006

Michel F. Jacques

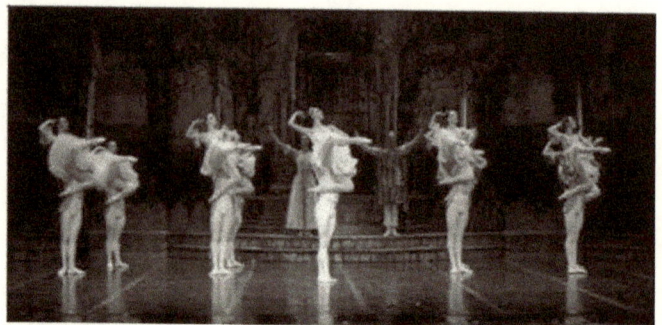

„Raymonda", year of 2007

Discussion

Every art has its own action field. The power of the arts' rule is in the irreplaceability of the means by which they affect over the audience. In the territory of ballet art, that is the dance. Dance is the strongest matter of expressing ballet as an art. "The character of the action of any art over the viewer or listener is determined by the whole complex of its expressive means, along with its specificity. The existence of dance would not be necessary if the content over which it rules could be expressed by painting, music or speech". (Г. Добровольская, „Танец Пантомима Балет", „Искусство", Ленинградское отделение, 1975, стр.124)

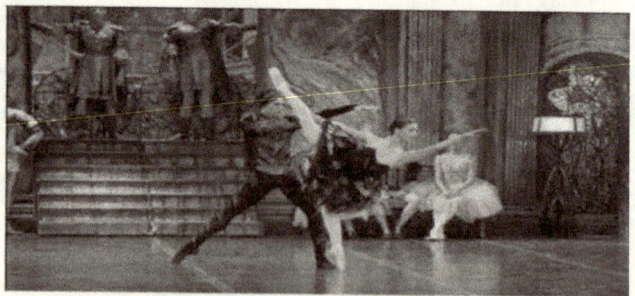

M. Pop Alexsova, D. Chebotar in „Swan lake"

Choreology Basic

From the Macedonian ballet stage review repertoire, the author concludes that skipping the rich possibilities of the dance does not go in the direction of improving the quality of the ballet performances.

In the synthetic ballet performance, the elements that contributes to the expression of an artistic idea are music, costume design, scenery, script, light design, but the main word belongs to choreography. Ignoring the potential of dance is unthinkable, and our practice confirms that performances in which dance is less represented do not last long in the ballet scene.

The dance-plastic shaping of the artistic imagination is the desired quality that moves ballet art in the right direction of development. Ballet can only really exist in its crystallized essential manifestations, not by the use of other expressive means of other arts.

Dance has its own sources of power that are dominant and through which plastic intonations are extracted, processed and organized by human movements. Dance "organizes the elements of plastic intonation (the body speaks and sings too), scattered in gestures, posture and manner of walking, to the extent the crescendo emotional excitement on a level that gets special character incarnated in measured, artistic proportioned complex movements – in a form ". (Б.Асафьев) И.Глебов, Театр русской Испании-„Театр",1923, № 2, стр.17)

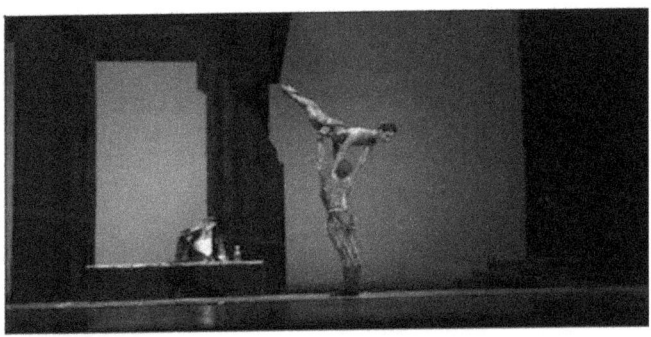

M. Pop Alexova, B.Kovachevsky in „Samson and Dalila", in 2012

Michel F. Jacques

In the book "In honor of dance" the author J. Slonimski emphasizes that: "The highest form of dramatic expression in a ballet performance - is the expression of dance. If it doesn't have that in it 'the soul flies'; leaving the stage with figures of living puppets with a demonstration of learned movements, aspiring to express something but remaining not clear and understandable. The idea comes to the ballet viewers attention and conqueres only when it is dressed in an artistic character - a dance character. The most current and content filled themes in ballet performance are forceless to act on us unless they are not transformed into choreographic characters. "(Ю. Слонимский, „В честь танца", „Искусство", Москва, 1968, стр.67,68)

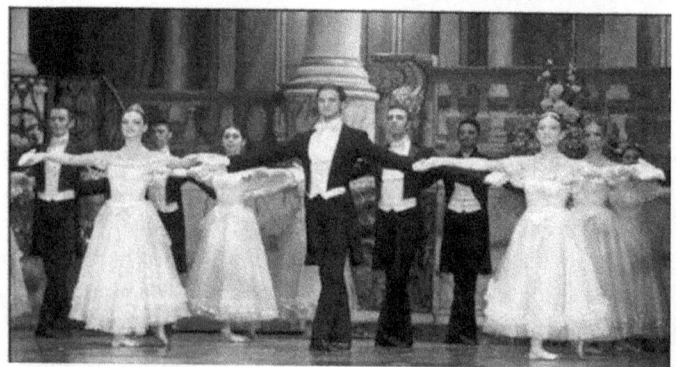

„Lady of the Camellias", year of 2014

The quote highlights the stage truth about ballet performance dance. Through a choreographic characters, its able to express the barely noticeable nuances of human mood, survival. Just to recall on the Greek philosopher Aristotle's statement "The game ... embodies the invisible thought."

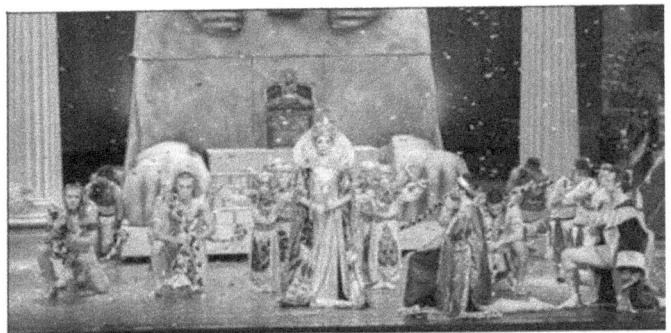

A.Miyalkova in „Cleopatra", year of 2016

Purpose

The purpose of the research goes on behalf the deposited material to provide a reason for scientific thought of nature and choreographic art development problems, to open professional discussions on the paths of development of national ballet art.

Methods

The method which is used represents a historical correlation analysis in terms of setted repertoire works on the stage of the National Theater of Opera and Ballet in Skopje.

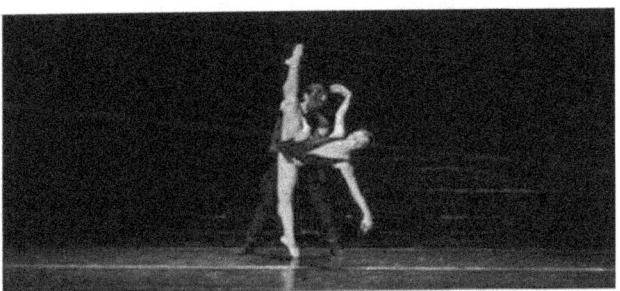

„Metamorphosis", year of 2018

Michel F. Jacques

Conclusion

The four periods which are considered in the history of ballet art at the National Opera and Ballet Theater in the Republic of North Macedonia have their distinctive features given in their titles. We can say for sure that ballet art is an integral part of our people's culture.

The question which arises is - What is the right path for the development of ballet art?

1. The author of the researched material, 70 years of ballet art in the Republic of North Macedonia, stands for the idea that the ballet performance, in the true sense of the word, in a national theater, should respect the laws on which the ballet heritage rests. "Among other things, traditions and innovations are not two antagonistic processes, but two sides of a process, unseparable sides. The innovation doesn't mean to terminate a tradition, it is not a substitution of one with the other, but a traditions developer, transforming them from within " (Ю. Слонимский, „В честь танца", „Искусство", Москва, 1968, стр.171)

Today as in the past, the problem of finding new contemporary solutions in ballet art had existed and has been resolved in one way or another. The best example for approaching new expression solutions is the ballet art reformation performed by the composer Petar Ilich Tchaikovsky.

Tchaikovsky does not disturb the already created forms and expressive means in the classical heritage. He remains faithful to the ballet forms (solo variation, duet, pas-de-deux, grand pas, and other forms) as well as the expressive means in ballet like (classical dance, character dance, ballroom dance, pantomime).

The reformation lies in the way of thinking, expressed through the musical symphony. The symphony music is part of the dance itself and requires from the choreographer to deeply penetrate into the meaning of music.

Choreology Basic

2. The second conclusion comes from the fact that in the setting of ballet performances, classical dance is often used as a basis. Domestic choreographers refresh the classics with national color. Remaining consistent with its principles, the classical dance, constantly renews its apparel with new sophisticated forms of expressing the modern day.

3. The deep insight into the very essence of dance is the third feature that the author longs for in matter of future development of ballet art. Great pedagogue of the 20th century Agripina Vaganova in the preface to her book says: "The classical heritage that we preserved is not determined by the technique. The shapes perfection is the greatest beauty of old ballets. To manage this perfection, to understand the character of the classical dance - it's an interesting task". (A.Vaganova, "Osnova klasicnog baleta", "Znanje", Belgrade, 1949, p.3)

Along the lucid insight into the nature of dance, the future of ballet lies solely in the hands of its dancers, pedagogues and choreographers.

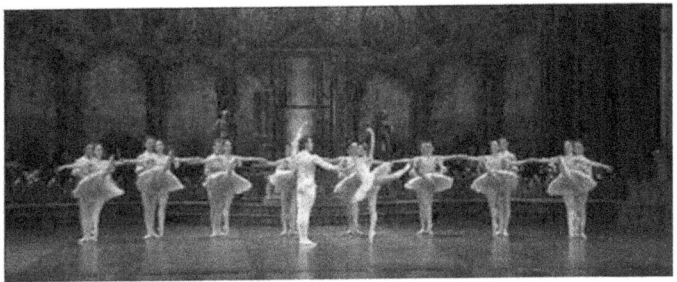

M.Kichevska-Shokarovska, Boban Kovachevski in „Raymonda"

Literature

1. (Б.Асафьев) И.Глебов, Театр русской Испании-„Театр",№ 2,1923

2. Г.Добровольская,,,Танец Пантомима Балет",,,Искусство",Ленинградское отделение, 1975

3. Федор Лопухов, „Хореографические откровенности" ,,,Искусство", 1972

4. Ю. Слонимский, „В честь танца", „Искусство", Москва, 1968

5. A.Vaganova, "Osnova klasicnog baleta", "Znanje", Belgrade, 1949

Ph.D Snezhana Filipovska (Cyrillic: Снежана Филиповска)

EDUCATION

In 1973 student at the State Institute for Theatrical Arts in Moscow.
In 1978 through special decision of the State Examination Commission - Master of Arts -as pedagogue - teacher – ballet master- (under the supervision of people artist of Russia,

Raissa Struchkova).

Upon the recommendation of the Council of Russian Theatrical Academy in 1993, she have received the title Ph.D. in Arts Science.

WORKING EXPERIENCE

Since 1970 soloist in the Ballet Company at the Macedonian National Theater.

In 1993 -1997 an Artistic Director of the Ballet Company at the Macedonian Opera and Ballet Theatre.

Working with international choreographers as an assistant choreographer in preparation of classical ballet productions: "Swan Lake", "Gisele", "La

Bajadere", "Sylphides", "Le Corsaire", "Don Quixote", "Legend of love", "Esmeralda", "Scheherazade".

As a dancer, I performed soloist roles in classical ballets "Gisele", "Don Quixote", "Sylphides", "Mirandolina", "Dance of Cadets", Pas de Trois in "Swan Lake", and in many nationals and modern ballets.

As a Choreographer setting up my own choreographies in many ballet plays, as well as in the following operas: "Aida", "Eugenie Onegin", "Ball under the masks" etc.

PEDAGOGUE WORK

I have experience in teaching all levels of professional students in classical ballet technique, pointe, variations and classical repertory, as well as character dance and history of ballet art. My teaching class is based on the method of classical exercises which is used in world known ballet schools in Russia. It is based on a Vaganova syllabus for the academic ballet education. The education and the experience of working with leading teachers in The Russian Theatrical Academy in Moscow allows me to apply an important principles that are fundamental of teaching dance and another professional ballet subjects throughout the world. With great respect and love, to my professors, I pass down the key traditions of training.

TEACHING EXPERIENCE

2010-Present - Associate professor at the Faculty of Music on Cyril and Methodius University in Skopje, Republic of North Macedonia, teaching following subjects:

History of ballet art

Duet dance

Composition of classical ballet

Michel F. Jacques

BOOK PUBLICATIONS

1. "History of the world of ballet"
2. "Founders of Macedonian ballet"
3. "Entries for the great masters of ballet"
4. "70 years of ballet art in Macedonia"

PROFESSIONAL MEMBERSHIPS

Active member (Academic) of the World Academy Plato

Member of the CID under registration number 27166 starting from year of 2019

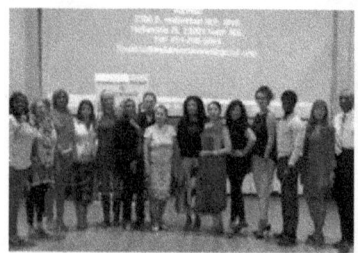
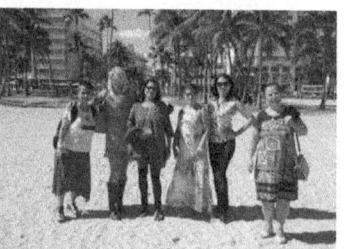
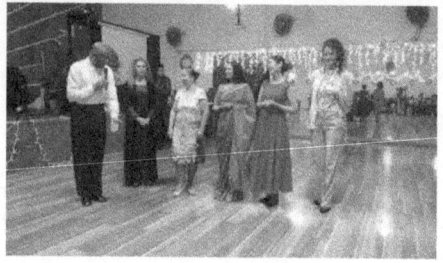

TABLE OF CONTENTS

Basics

What is Dance ....
Why People Dance...
Musicology & Choreology ....
Levels of a professional dancer.
Dancing Tips ....

Types of Dances

Latin/Rhythm..
Ballroom/Smooth..

Elements of Dance

Musical Counts & Beat Value....................................NA
Tempo..NA
Direction..NA

Smooth Dances

Foxtrot ....NA
Tango ....NA
Slow Waltz ....NA
Vienna Waltz ....NA

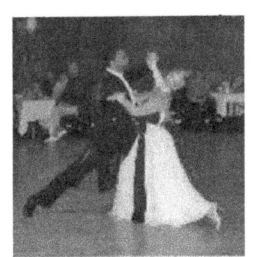

Rhythm Dances

Rumba .... NA
Chachacha .... NA
Mambo/Salsa .... NA
Samba .... NA
Swing .... NA
Disco/Hustle .... NA
Konpa .... NA
Bolero .... N/A
Merengue................................

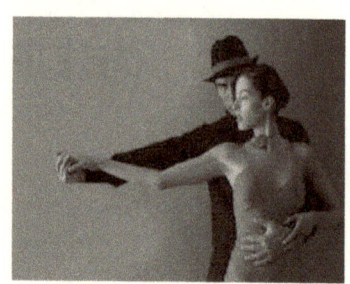

The Three Families of Dance
Social Ballroom Dancing
By Randy Pittman

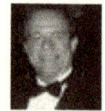

The Three Families of Social Ballroom dance; Smooth, Latin and Swing. Today's Ballroom dance organizations use two divisions in dance. ISTD (Imperial Society of Teachers of Dancing) the International style of dance, divide dance with the terms, Standard and Latin. NDCA (National Dance Council of America) the American style of dance, divide dance with into Smooth and Rhythm. Using only two divisions for dance is inadequate. In the ISTD, the dance of jive is included in the Latin division. Jive is not a Latin dance; it is a swing dance. The NDCA Rhythm section includes Cha Cha Cha, Rumba, Swing, Mambo, and Bolero. These are Latin dances not Rhythm dances. In my opinion, Rhythm is a musical term not a dance category. The Swing is not a Latin or Rhythm dance. Therefore, the Swing family of dance needs to be created. The swing family has always been present, just not highlighted. The Swing family of dance includes; Jive, Triple time Swing (East Coast Swing), Single time Swing, Lindy Hop, West Coast Swing, Hustle and Shag. This is the Swing family of dance. The International and American Standard of dance, I love and respect. What the Ballroom dance world has done to develop and grow ballroom dance, has been amazing. Now it is time to expand and properly divide the world of dance, the three families of social ballroom dance, Smooth, Latin and Swing.

What is Dance?

Dance - The architecture of all human movements, which is dancing to the equivalence of music; the interpretation of music, Interpersonal communication.

Posture – The genetic and cultural heritage; no two people have the same posture; There are as many postures as there are people.

Dance is the equivalence of music

In order to translate a language to a certain level, you must learn the new language at that level. If choreology is the equivalence of Music

Why People Dance .... NA

Musical & Choreography .... NA

Levels of Dance .... NA

Dancing Tips .... NA

Michel F. Jacques

Why People should learn how to dance?

The Benefits of Dancing

1. To enjoy and please your partner	11. To establish communication ("marriage") between a lady and man	21. A sense of achievement or Accomplishment
2. To satisfy and entertain the audience		22. A release of tensions
3. To make a good living (for money)	12. More Fun and Enjoyment out of life	23. Ease and assurance socially
4. To earn a title	13. Increasing Self-confidence	24. A hobby or interest
5. To compete for yourself, school, city, state, country, be famous etc.	14. Meeting people and Making Friends	25. A means of expression
	15. Becoming happier	26. Admiration of others
6. Better health and physical benefits	16. Self-Improvement	27. Recreation of entertainment
7. Improved social life	18. Attending and Enjoying more parties	28. Increased conversational ability
8. Relaxation	19. Business reasons	29. Increased popularity
9. Exercise	20. Acquiring more grace and pose	30. Perform in exhibitions
10. Improved appearance		31. Social teaching
		32. Overcoming shyness And Etiquettes

Musicology & Choreology

Musicology – The science of creating, construct & arranging music.

Choreology – The science of movement (graphic design of the feet, foot point.)

Choreography – The art of creating sophisticated movement; philosophy, it is an art.

Choreology – The architecture of all human movements (graphic design of your feet)

- Dance as if you were drawing on the dance floor with your feet

- A dancer uses the dance floor to create blue point, as a writer would use a piece of paper to calculate his blue point in building constructions.

- The elements in choreographic works like the 26 letters of the alphabet.

- *Amalgamation - The art or process of combining, merging or uniting dance movements.

Let's Dance.

Musicology = Choreology

Choreology	Musicology
• Footwork • Foot Position- There are a total of 5 • Alignment-Our Body position according to the Room using accurate amount of turns. • Amount of Turns: 1/8, 2/8, 3/8, 4/8 etc. • Every room has 8 positions; each wall has 4 corners, Floor Craft. Traveling Direction... • Dance position – Your body position according to your partner. Using proper posture, accurate amount of resistance using for perfect Leading and following. Communication between a Gentleman and a lady Moving on the dance floor as a Couple.	**The 5 Elements of Music:** 1. Rhythm – The specific sound within music that sounds the same from beginning to end and it is never changes. 2. Tempo – How fast or slow the music is playing. 3. Count or Beat Value – All music has 4 main beats in a bar/measure; the Waltz is an exception, which has 3 main beats. 4. BPM – Bars per Minute MPM – Measure per minute. 5. High and Low – high is a note an upbeat and the low is the downbeat
Dancing Tips Men usually start on their left foot Lady usually start on their right foot, The direction of your head over the left elbow in close facing position.	• Syncopated Beats- usually lasts the time to say "and" the space in between each main beat; 1 & 2 & 3 & 4 &. • Each dance has different way to count the beats.

Levels in the Mastery of Dance:

Effective for Health Care Practitioners

Bronze = College Degree
Silver = Bachelor's degree
Gold = Master's degree
Gold Bar = P.H.D. level

Types of Dance Categories

Rhythm and Smooth = American Latin and Standard = International	Rhythm Dances = American cultural dance style Smooth Dances = American Ballroom
Latin /Rhythm Dances	**Standard/Smooth Dances**
Cha-cha Rumba Meringue/Konpa Bolero Mambo/Salsa Samba Swing Disco/Hustle Jive	Slow Waltz Tango Foxtrot Viennese Waltz Quickstep

Each dance has a way to count the beats. Downbeat = 1st & 4th beat in some Dances.

Dance characteristics based on the basic Rhythm of the Music.

Characteristics of dance change on the basic rhythm or changes in tempo of the music.

Latin/Rhythm

In Latin dances, our toe is the first part of our foot that must touch the dance floor. "Cha-Cha is the first dance you learn, if you don't know the cha-cha-cha, it may come harder to dance Mambo/Salsa on the 2. So, learn the cha-cha-cha.

Ballroom/Smooth

There is a total of five dances in the Smooth category. In Smooth dances, the heel is the first part of our foot that must touch the dance floor.

Cha-cha

The Cha-cha-cha dance originated in Cuba. It is the first Rhythm dance in the ballroom style dance category that is commonly performed in dancing competitions. It is usually known as the basic for all Afro-Cuban dances

Rumba

Known in the United States as the Rumba is a composite of several dances popular in Cuba, including the **guaracha**, the Haitian **bolero**, the **Cuban son**, and all have similar rhythms that can be traced to religious and ceremonial dances of Africa.

Merengue

The Merengue is the national dance of the Dominican Republic and, to some extent, it originated of the island neighbor Haiti. Merengue has existed since the early years of the Dominican Republic, around the time of the Spanish-American War (1898). There are many versions and interpretations of the origins of Merengue.

Michel F. Jacques

Samba

Samba developed in Brazil, samba owes its rhythm and moves to the African slaves danced on the Brazilian sugarcane plantations. The traditional African 2/4 percussive beat, once slavery ended, the dancers migrated outside of cities, where they put together dance troupes for *carnival*. Today, it would be impossible to imagine *carnival* without samba in Brazil.

The Swing

The swing is an American cultural dance, dates to the 1920's, where the black community danced to contemporary Jazz music, discovered the Charleston and the Lindy Hop. The style of Swing popular in the New York Savoy Ballroom in the 30's and 40's originally danced to Swing music. The Savoy style of swing is a very fast, bouncing, casual-looking style of dancing. The true characteristic is of the swing is bouncing action.

Disco/Hustle

Disco/Hustle Originated in United States as a free style dance. The Hustle is believed to have developed in New York in 1970, with line dances for groups of people and partnership dances. There two type of Disco/Hustle, the 3 counts and the 4 counts. Fourth count Hustle is similar to Ballroom meringue/konpa dancing.

The Foxtrot

The Fox-trot originated in New York. Harry Fox was doing trotting steps to ragtime music, and people referred to his dance as "Fox's Trot." The Foxtrot was the most significant dance in all of ballroom dancing. There is multiple type of rhythm in the fox-trot dance, and in some ways, it is very complex and the hardest dance to learn!

The Mambo

Mambo originated in Haiti back in the late 1800, developed as a dance form in Cuba. Back home in Haiti, 'Mambo' means a voodoo priestess who performs the rituals of witchdoctor while dancing. The music of Mambo is a blend of the cha-cha of Afro-Cuban music. It was Perez Prado, who introduced the dance in a night-club in Havana, then USA in 1940s. It becomes an old generation name for Salsa.

The Waltz

The Waltz is the oldest of the ballroom dances. Waltz danced to a 3/4-time music; accent is on the first beat of the music. (To advance easily and successfully). Waltz originated in the suburbs of Vienna and in the alpine region of Austria and Germany, dating from the middle of the sixteenth Century. The dance style imported to the United States. It was in the United States the two new forms of the waltz developed, the Boston, which was a slower form as compared to the Viennese waltz.

Tango

The Tango brought to Argentina by African Slaves. Today it is the most Romantic and fascinating of all dances, developed in Buenos Aires for couples. Tango is one of the easiest of the ballroom dance to learn. There are 3 categories of tango, the American style, the International style and Argentinian style. Each of these styles is a social dance, however International Style is generally often used in ballroom dance sport competitions.

Konpa

THE MUSIC & THE DANCE – "A WAY OF LIVING"

Konpa, is a music derived from African and European roots influenced by Mambo, Chachacha of Cuba, the Meringue of Dominican Republic and Samba of Brazil.

Like the Argentinian tango style, in Konpa couples dance very close together. when they are in ballroom position in contrast to Salsa styles.

Couples dance with smaller steps, one bent knee, and lower to the ground naturally generating good hip movement. They also are not shy in moving their bodies, shoulders, legs and feet from side to side and diagonal.

In KONPA, like in club dancing, couples often break apart for a time to groove on their own when the music goes into a heavy percussion and bass breakdown riff. This trend has connections with typical African dance, Afro-Cuban ceremonial dances, and American Swing or Rock N-Roll.

Like in mambo, casino dancing, as the rhythm gets faster, there is a tendency in Konpa for men to take the "star" role and challenge each other as they show off their best moves, change partners, dance in circle creating a high-spirited experience.

The Music gives Ballroom dancers the opportunity to do chachacha, Salsa, samba, disco hustle, swing & meringue.

THE HISTORY "of THE MUSIC OF PEACE"

In 1950's Nemours Jean Baptiste Band and the dancing community invented konpa direct which became Konpa in late 60s as a social music & dance form to restore in Haiti the true social democracy. From an historical and logical perspective, Nemours teamed up with virtuous saxophonist Weber Sicot and other great musicians to conceive the Konpa Music. Both Nemours and Sicot are to Konpa what Beethoven and Mozart are to classical music. They were the national icons and idols of the first black independent republic in the world.

The transition from Haitian folklore to Konpa was not easy. The early history of Konpa (Compas) began with the formation of big band orchestras and folkloric groups in the 1940's and 1950's. The

Choreology Basic

greatest competition for Nemours and Sicot were Les Jazz Des Jeunes, Septentrional and Tropicana of which the latter are two of the oldest Haitian bands, which are still active today.

This period also marked the beginning of ballroom dance in Haiti. During this time, number of Haitian musicians like Nemours, Sicot, Charles Dessalines, Gerard Dupervil, Michel Desgrottes, Richard Duroseau, Joe Trouillot, Raroule Guillaume, Ti Paris, and of course the greatest Haitian conga player of all time (Tambourineur) TI RORO, struggled to find their own musical identity.

They could be found playing all styles of Jazz, Rumba, Jazz, Bolero, Meringue and Salsa etc. One of the music styles you can use to dance all Latin rhythm. The hitting wave of the Mini-Jazz movement with small bands pairing electric guitars, electric bass, drums, percussion, keyboard and saxophone started in the mid 1960's launched by Haitian youth from Port-au-Prince gave birth to a totally different and commercial sound of Kompa.

Today Konpa music is a huge new brand worldwide thanks to the remarkable efforts of legends Magnum Band, Les Skah Shah, Le Scorpio, Bossa Combo, Raoul Denis jr, that formed the core of this middle-class popular music movement.

Tabou Combo is the first Haitian band to garner acclaim after its 1969 album that incorporated major influences from American Funk. By 1984, Tabou Combo had become an international sensation playing its chart-topping hits to stadiums in Paris and around the globe.

In the History of Music, Konpa is the tool Haiti has earned to Communicate, Educate and Promote the True cultural identity of the people. I have worked for the past 30 years as an Architect of human movement, to create the concept of learning the konpa. Introduced to the International dance Council/Unesco and the world dance sports organizations. I am Proud to be able to represent in this volume the ballroom Konpa Dance art Forms of Haiti.

Rhythm Dance	Count (the basic/primary rhythm)
Cha-cha or Cha-cha-cha	2,3-4 & 1 - (2, 3) Rock step or Rocking step - (4 & 1) The time to express the "Cha-cha-cha" (side together side)
Rumba	1,2; 3,4 or 3, 4; 1, 2 (quick, quick, slow); start on 3,4; To set characteristic of the Rumba, pause between 1, 2 so three steps are done in four beats;
Swing	1 & 2, 3 & 4, 5, 6 (basic movement is done within the six beats; American Cultural behavior)
Bolero	(Also moves in a different direction) 1,2; 3,4 or 3, 4; 1, 2 slow quick, quick or (quick, quick, slow); start on 3,4; To set the characteristic of the bolero, pause between 1, 2 so three steps are done in four beats.
Mambo/Salsa	2, 3, 4 & 1(same as cha-cha but you hold 4&1; there are 4 beats per bar) with a breaking action on the second beat of the music. It's ok to break on 1
Samba	1 & 2, 3 & 4 (characteristic is a bouncing action) like playing basketball.
Hustle	&, 1, 2, 3
Konpa	& & 1, 2, 3, 4

Smooth Dance	Count (the basic/Primary Rhythm)
Waltz "Slow Waltz"	& 1,2,3, & 1, 2, 3 (or & 1, 2, 3, & 4, 5, 6); uses 3/4 time
Tango	& & 1, 2, 3, 4, & & 5,6,7,8 (there are multiple syncopated beats preceding the 1st beat); slow, slow, quick, quick, slow.
Viennese Waltz "Fast Waltz"	& 1, 2, 3; & 1, 2, 3 (or 1,2,3,4,5,6; same count as slow waltz but faster)
Foxtrot Quickstep	1, 2, 3, 4, 5, 6 - 1, 2, 3, 4, 5, 6 (slow-slow, quick-quick, slow-slow, quick-quick); Count for the primary (basic) rhythm. There is one low and one high (two distinct sounds) 1st beat is always on the low. Fox-trot has 4 types of rhythm to be concerned with. Primary, Secondary, Straight and syncopated.

(American Style Latin) Rhythm Dance Positions!
Closed Facing, Open Facing, outside partner Left & Right, Shadow left & right, Left & right side by side, C.B.M.

Hustle Merengue	Samba Konpa	Cha-Cha Mambo	Rumba	Bolero	East Coast Swing
Closed Facing or double-handhold open facing Position.	Latin closed-facing position Or Open-Facing Position	Latin closed-facing position Or Open-Facing Position	Latin closed facing Or Open-Facing Position	Latin closed-facing position Or Open-Facing Position	Open-facing or closed-facing position with men's left/ woman's right hand at the hip height

American Style Smooth Dance Position

Slow Waltz & Viennese Waltz	Foxtrot	Tango	Peabody
Smooth closed-facing position	Smooth closed-facing position	Smooth closed-facing position; Man, torso in ⅛ right turn & Lady torso in ⅛ left turn; knees decently bent	Smooth closed-facing position

Modern Names	Which Dance You Refer To	Old generation Names
Salsa	Over age of 50	Mambo
Quickstep	Over age of 70	Peabody

* If you are under the age of 50, you may call the dances by their modern names: Salsa, Bachata, Zouk or Boogy-Woogy.

Elements of Dance

There are **three** ways to teach dance steps to any student:

Count - gives the right beat value; you need to know which beat is the 1, the 2, the 3, and the 4.

Tempo - gives the speed of the movement as referred to the speed of the music.

Slow, slow, quick, quick etc.

Direction – gives where you go; For example, back, forward, side, together, side etc.; deals with the graphic design of footwork

Smooth Dances

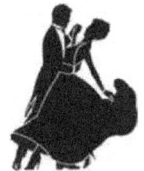
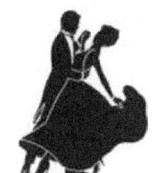

Fox-trot

Characteristics:

- In the Smooth dances, you take forward steps heel first
- And you take back steps toe first
- 1st beat is always on the low or down
- This dance is with straight line position; there is no rising or falling

Count: 1-2, 3-4, 5-6; 1-2, 3-4, 5-6 (1st beat is always on the low).

The 4 Rhythms of the Fox-trot:
1. Primary Rhythm - slow, slow, quick-quick
2. Secondary Rhythm – Slow, quick, quick.
3. Straight Rhythm - slow, slow, slow or Quick, Quick, Quick
4. Syncopated – slow, quick & quick & slow

Michel F. Jacques

American Social Dance Syllabus Fox-Trot

Bronze I	I FP T L/F S C	**Student Variations**
1. Forward Basic	☐ ☐ ☐ ☐ ☐ ☐	
2. Promenade	☐ ☐ ☐ ☐ ☐ ☐	
3. Magic Left Turn	☐ ☐ ☐ ☐ ☐ ☐	
Amalgamations:		

Bronze II

4. Promenade Pivot ☐ ☐ ☐ ☐ ☐ ☐		
5. Quater Turns ☐ ☐ ☐ ☐ ☐ ☐ 6. Swing Step		
Amalgamations:		

Bronze III

7. Spiral ☐ ☐ ☐ ☐ ☐ ☐		
8. Simple Twinkle ☐ ☐ ☐ ☐ ☐ ☐		
9. Triple Twinkle Closed ☐ ☐ ☐ ☐ ☐ ☐		
Amalgamations:		

Choreology Basic

Bronze IV

10. Open Twinkle ☐ ☐ ☐ ☐ ☐ ☐	
11. Closed Passing twinkle ☐ ☐ ☐ ☐ ☐ ☐ --- 12. Open Passing twinkle	

amalgamations:

I (Introduction) **FP** (Foot Positions) **T** (Timing) **L/F** (Lead &Follow) S (Style) C (Checked)

American Social Dance Syllabus Tango
Elementary SCHOOL FIGURES

Student VARIATIONS

Bronze I   **I FP T L/F S C**

1. **Basic**							
2. **Corte & Lift**							
3. **Promenade**							
Amalgamations:							

Bronze II

4. **Promenade Flare**						
5. **Rock-N-Fans** ---------------------------- 6. **Rock-N-Corte**						

Michel F. Jacques

Amalgamations:

Bronze III

7. Promenade Pivots							
8. Grapevine Check & Fans 9. Promenade Ronde							

Amalgamations:

Tango Bronze IV Student Variations

10. Reverse Left-N-Outside Swivel							
11. Double Fans 12. Shadow Rock & Fan							
Amalgamations:							
I (Introduction) **FP** (Foot Positions) **T** (Timing) **L/F** (Lead &Follow) **S** (Style) **C** (Checked)							

Characteristics:

- Forward steps are taken heel first

Count: & & 1, 2, 3, 4,5,6,7,8 (there are multiply syncopated beats preceding the 1st beat); slow, slow, quick, quick, slow;
Pictures

Slow Waltz

American Social Dance Syllabus

Elementary SCHOOL FIGURES

S. Waltz: Bronze I   **I FP T L/F S C**   **tudent Variations**

1. Box/Turning ☐ ☐ ☐ ☐ ☐ ☐	
2. Under arm turn ☐ ☐ ☐ ☐ ☐ ☐	
3. 2 Ways Hesitations ☐ ☐ ☐ ☐ ☐ ☐	
Amalgamations:	

Bronze II

4. Spiral ☐ ☐ ☐ ☐ ☐ ☐	
5. Spiral Developee ☐ ☐ ☐ ☐ ☐ ☐	
6. Simple Twinkle ☐ ☐ ☐ ☐ ☐ ☐	
Amalgamations:	

Bronze III

7. Closed Triple Twinkle ☐ ☐ ☐ ☐ ☐ ☐	
8. Open Triple Twinkle ☐ ☐ ☐ ☐ ☐ ☐	
9. Promenade Chasse ☐ ☐ ☐ ☐ ☐ ☐	
Amalgamations:	

Bronze IV

9. Reverse left Turn ☐ ☐ ☐ ☐ ☐ ☐
10. Close PassingTwinkle ☐ ☐ ☐ ☐ ☐ ☐
11. Open Passing Twinkle ☐ ☐ ☐ ☐ ☐ ☐
12. Reverse Right turn ☐ ☐ ☐ ☐ ☐ ☐
Amalgamations:
I (Introduction) **FP** (Foot Positions) **T** (Timing) **L/F** (Lead &Follow) S (Style) C (Checked)

Characteristics: Rising and Fall: Forward steps are taken heel first
Count: & 1,2,3, & 1, 2, 3 (or & 1, 2, 3, & 4, 5, 6); uses ¾ time

Slow Waltz vs. Foxtrot

Slow Waltz has a rising and falling action.	Couple starts lowing at the end of the 3rd beat of the Music, Step on 1& start rise at the end of the first beat continue rise on 2 up to the third beat and lower…

Rhythm Dances

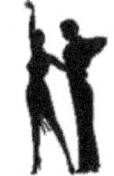

Rumba

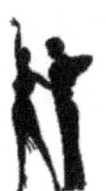

Characteristics:

- Forward and back step are taken with toe first
- In the Rumba you pause between 1, 2 so three steps are done in four beats;
- In the Rumba you start on 3,4 quick, quick or 1,2 (slow)

Count: 1,2; 3,4 or 3, 4; 1, 2 (Slow, quick, quick, or Quick, Quick, slow.

Foxtrot vs. Rumba

The Foxtrot	The Rumba
1. Has no hip movement	1. Has hip movement
2. Heel is the first to touch the floor in forward step.	2. Toe is the first part of foot to touch the floor in forward step.
3. Both feet meet at the four corners of the basic box.	3. Both feet meet only at two corners of the basic box.
4. Tempo: Slow, Slow, Quick, Quick	4. Tempo: Quick, Quick, Slow

Michel F. Jacques

American Social Dance Syllabus

RUMBA

Elementary SCHOOL FIGURES   Student VARIATIONS

Bronze I   I FP T L/F S C

1. Rumba Box (Basic)	☐ ☐ ☐ ☐ ☐ ☐	
2. Parallel break	☐ ☐ ☐ ☐ ☐ ☐	
3. Under Arm turn	☐ ☐ ☐ ☐ ☐ ☐	
Amalgamations:	☐ ☐ ☐ ☐ ☐ ☐	

Bronze II

4. Cross over break	☐ ☐ ☐ ☐ ☐ ☐	
5. Peek A Boo	☐ ☐ ☐ ☐ ☐ ☐	
6. Cross body -Lead	☐ ☐ ☐ ☐ ☐ ☐	
Amalgamations.	☐ ☐ ☐ ☐ ☐ ☐	

Bronze III

7. 5th Position Break ☐ ☐ ☐ ☐ ☐ ☐	
8. Sweet Heart ☐ ☐ ☐ ☐ ☐ ☐	
9. Cross-over swivel ☐ ☐ ☐ ☐ ☐ ☐	
Amalgamations:	
Bronze IV 10. Open Cuban Walk & U.A.T ☐ ☐ ☐ ☐ ☐ ☐	
11. Promenade Ronde ☐ ☐ ☐ ☐ ☐ ☐	
---	
12. Half-moon ☐ ☐ ☐ ☐ ☐ ☐	
Amalgamations:	
I (Introduction) **FP** (Foot Positions) **T** (Timing) **L/F** (Lead &Follow) S (Style) C (Checked)	

Choreology Basic

Cha-Cha-Cha

American Social Dance Syllabus

CHA-CHA
Elementary SCHOOL FIGURES   Student VARIATIONS

Bronze I   **I FP T L/F S C**

1. Basic	☐ ☐ ☐ ☐ ☐ ☐	
2. Parallel Break	☐ ☐ ☐ ☐ ☐ ☐	
3. Open Break & U.A.T	☐ ☐ ☐ ☐ ☐ ☐	
Amalgamations:	☐ ☐ ☐ ☐ ☐ ☐	

Bronze II

4 Cross Over U.A.T	☐ ☐ ☐ ☐ ☐ ☐	
5. Cross Body Lead	☐ ☐ ☐ ☐ ☐ ☐	
6. 5th Position Break	☐ ☐ ☐ ☐ ☐ ☐	
Amalgamations:		

Bronze III

7. Cross Over Swivel	☐ ☐ ☐ ☐ ☐ ☐	
8. Pee-K-Boo	☐ ☐ ☐ ☐ ☐ ☐	
9. Progressive Lock ☐	☐ ☐ ☐ ☐ ☐ ☐	
Amalgamations:		

Cha cha Cha Bronze IV

10. Sweet Heart	☐ ☐ ☐ ☐ ☐ ☐	
11. Half-moon.	☐ ☐ ☐ ☐ ☐ ☐	
_____		
12. The Snaps	☐ ☐ ☐ ☐ ☐ ☐	
Amalgamations:		
I (Introduction) **FP** (Foot Positions) **T** (Timing) L/**F** (Lead &Follow) S (Style) C (Checked)		

Forward and back step are taken with toe first
- (2, 3) Rock step or Rocking step
- (4 & 1) the time to express the "Cha-cha-cha"
Count: 2,3,4 & 1

American Social Dance Syllabus
Konpa

Elementary SCHOOL FIGURES　　　　Students VARIATIONS
Bronze I　　　　**I FP T L/F S C**

1. 4 ways Basic ☐ ☐ ☐ ☐ ☐ ☐	
2. Rotating Basic ☐ ☐ ☐ ☐ ☐ ☐	
3.Promenade ☐ ☐ ☐ ☐ ☐ ☐	
Amalgamations:	

Bronze II

4.Open Promenade ☐ ☐ ☐ ☐ ☐ ☐ (5th Position)	
5.U.A.T Right & left ☐ ☐ ☐ ☐ ☐ ☐	
6. Cross Body Lead ☐ ☐ ☐ ☐ ☐ ☐	
Amalgamations:	

Choreology Basic

Bronze III

7 Promenade Scallop ☐ ☐ ☐ ☐ ☐ ☐	
8. Wrap In & Out ☐ ☐ ☐ ☐ ☐ ☐ 9. Over the Shoulder Turn ☐ ☐ ☐ ☐ ☐ ☐	
Amalgamations:	

Bronze IV

10. Whap in & CircularTurn ☐ ☐ ☐ ☐ ☐ ☐	
11. Pretsel ☐ ☐ ☐ ☐ ☐ ☐ 12. La Kompasita ☐ ☐ ☐ ☐ ☐ ☐	
Amalgamation	

I (Introduction) **FP** (Foot Positions) **T** (Timing) **L/F** (Lead &Follow) S (Style) C (Checked)

American Style Viennese Waltz

Elementary SCHOOL FIGURES   Student VARIATIONS

Bronze I   **I FP T L/F S C**

1. Basic Forward & Back ☐ ☐ ☐ ☐ ☐ ☐	
2. Left & Right change ☐ ☐ ☐ ☐ ☐ ☐	
3. 4 ways **Hesitation** ☐ ☐ ☐ ☐ ☐ ☐	
Amalgamations:	

Bronze II

4. Open break ☐ ☐ ☐ ☐ ☐ ☐	
5. Reverse Left turn ☐ ☐ ☐ ☐ ☐ ☐	
6. Reverse right turn ☐ ☐ ☐ ☐ ☐ ☐	
Amalgamations:	

Michel F. Jacques

Bronze III

7. Open Break & U.A.T	☐ ☐ ☐ ☐ ☐ ☐	
8. Spiral Turn	☐ ☐ ☐ ☐ ☐ ☐	
9. Back Lock	☐ ☐ ☐ ☐ ☐ ☐	
Amalgamations:		

Bronze IV

10. **Simple Twinkle**	☐ ☐ ☐ ☐ ☐ ☐	
11 **Back Spot Turn**	☐ ☐ ☐ ☐ ☐ ☐	
12.**Spot Turn**	☐ ☐ ☐ ☐ ☐ ☐	
Amalgamations:		
I (Introduction) **FP** (Foot Positions) **T** (Timing) L/**F** (Lead &Follow) S (Style) C (Checked)		

American Social Dance Syllabus
East Coast Swing

Elementary SCHOOL FIGURES   Student VARIATIONS

Bronze I   **I FP T L/F S C**

1.Basic Rotation	☐ ☐ ☐ ☐ ☐ ☐	
2.Open Break/Separation	☐ ☐ ☐ ☐ ☐ ☐	
3.Lady's Right & Left turns	☐ ☐ ☐ ☐ ☐ ☐	
Amalgamations:		

Bronze II

4. Behind the back	☐ ☐ ☐ ☐ ☐ ☐	
5. The Points	☐ ☐ ☐ ☐ ☐ ☐	
6. Stop & Go	☐ ☐ ☐ ☐ ☐ ☐	
Amalgamations:		

Choreology Basic

Bronze III

7. Tuck in turn ☐ ☐ ☐ ☐ ☐ ☐	
8. Wrap In & Out ☐ ☐ ☐ ☐ ☐ ☐	
9. Over the Shoulder ☐ ☐ ☐ ☐ ☐ ☐	
Amalgamations:	

Bronze IV

10. Sliding Door ☐ ☐ ☐ ☐ ☐ ☐	
11. Shoulder Touch ☐ ☐ ☐ ☐ ☐ ☐	
12. Crazy leg ☐ ☐ ☐ ☐ ☐ ☐	
Amalgamations:	
I (Introduction) **FP** (Foot Positions) **T** (Timing) **L/F** (Lead &Follow) **S** (Style) **C** (Checked)	

American Social Dance Syllabus
Samba

Elementary SCHOOL FIGURES Student VARIATIONS

Bronze I   **I FP T L/F S C**

1. Basic Turning ☐ ☐ ☐ ☐ ☐ ☐	
2. Balancete (5th position) ☐ ☐ ☐ ☐ ☐ ☐	
3. Lady Right turns ☐ ☐ ☐ ☐ ☐ ☐	
Amalgamations:	

Bronze II

4. Copa Cabana ☐ ☐ ☐ ☐ ☐ ☐	
5. Throw out ☐ ☐ ☐ ☐ ☐ ☐	
6. Separation (open Break ☐ ☐ ☐ ☐ ☐ ☐	
Amalgamations:	

Bronze III

7. Cross lead ☐ ☐ ☐ ☐ ☐ ☐	
8. Spiral ☐ ☐ ☐ ☐ ☐ ☐	
9. Promenade Bota Fogo ☐ ☐ ☐ ☐ ☐ ☐	
Amalgamations:	

Bronze IV

10. 2 ways Compasso ☐ ☐ ☐ ☐ ☐ ☐	
11. Reverse Copa ☐ ☐ ☐ ☐ ☐ ☐	
12. Promenade runs ☐ ☐ ☐ ☐ ☐ ☐	
Amalgamations:	
I (Introduction) **FP** (Foot Positions) **T** (Timing) **L/F** (Lead &Follow) S (Style) C (Checked)	

American Social Dance Syllabus
BOLERO

Elementary SCHOOL FIGURES

Student VARIATIONS

Bronze I **I FP T L/F S C**

1. Bolero Basic ☐ ☐ ☐ ☐ ☐ ☐	
2. Under Arm Turn ☐ ☐ ☐ ☐ ☐ ☐ Right & Left (Lady)	
3. Cross Over Break ☐ ☐ ☐ ☐ ☐ ☐	
Amalgamations:	

Bronze II

4. Open Break U.A.T ☐ ☐ ☐ ☐ ☐ ☐	
5. Closed Cross Lead ☐ ☐ ☐ ☐ ☐ ☐	
6. Left Side pass (open) ☐ ☐ ☐ ☐ ☐ ☐	
Amalgamations:	

Choreology Basic

Bronze III

7. Right Side Pass	☐ ☐ ☐ ☐ ☐ ☐	
8. The Swivel	☐ ☐ ☐ ☐ ☐ ☐	
9. 5th position Break	☐ ☐ ☐ ☐ ☐ ☐	
Amalgamations:		

Bronze IV

10. Parallel Outside Swivel	☐ ☐ ☐ ☐ ☐ ☐	
11. Promenade Ronde	☐ ☐ ☐ ☐ ☐ ☐	
12. Traveling Cross	☐ ☐ ☐ ☐ ☐ ☐	
Amalgamations:		
I (Introduction) **FP** (Foot Positions) **T** (Timing) **L/F** (Lead &Follow) S (Style) C (Checked)		

MAMBO

American Social Dance Syllabus
Mambo

Elementary SCHOOL FIGURES Student VARIATIONS

Bronze I **I FP T L/F S C**

1. Basic	☐ ☐ ☐ ☐ ☐ ☐	
2. Side Break	☐ ☐ ☐ ☐ ☐ ☐	
3. Open Break & U.A.T	☐ ☐ ☐ ☐ ☐ ☐	
Amalgamations:		

Bronze II

4 Cross Over break & U.A.T	☐ ☐ ☐ ☐ ☐ ☐	
5. Cross Body Lead	☐ ☐ ☐ ☐ ☐ ☐	
6. 5th Position Break	☐ ☐ ☐ ☐ ☐ ☐	
Amalgamations:		

Bronze III

4 Cross Over break & U.A.T	☐ ☐ ☐ ☐ ☐ ☐	
5. Cross Body Lead	☐ ☐ ☐ ☐ ☐ ☐	
6. 5th Position Break	☐ ☐ ☐ ☐ ☐ ☐	
Amalgamations:		

7. Cross Over Swivel	☐ ☐ ☐ ☐ ☐ ☐	
8. Pee-K-Boo	☐ ☐ ☐ ☐ ☐ ☐	
9. The Towell	☐ ☐ ☐ ☐ ☐ ☐	
Amalgamations:		

Choreology Basic

Cha cha Cha Bronze IV

10. Sweet Heart	☐ ☐ ☐ ☐ ☐ ☐	
11. Half-moon.	☐ ☐ ☐ ☐ ☐ ☐	
12. Pretsel & Reverse turn	☐ ☐ ☐ ☐ ☐ ☐	
Amalgamations:		
I (Introduction) **FP** (Foot Positions) **T** (Timing) **L/F** (Lead &Follow) S (Style) C (Checked)		

Forward and back step are taken with toe first

- (2, 3) Rock step or Rocking step
- (4 & 1) the time to express the "Cha-cha-cha"

Count: 2,3,4 & 1

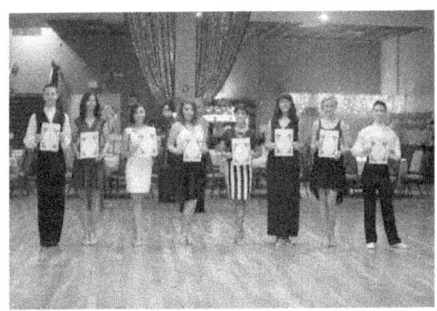

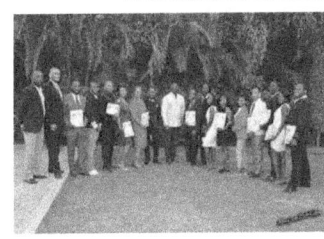
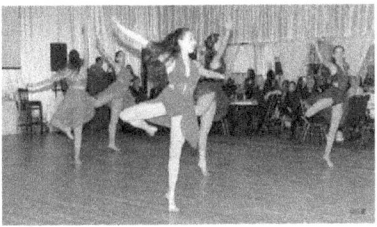

Michel F. Jacques

Bianca Munoz

My name is Bianca Marie Muñoz, and I am from Wellington, Florida. I am 17 years old and am currently in 12th grade at Sun coast Community High School. I was born on May 5, 1996, in Geneva Illinois, a suburb about 40 minutes outside of Downtown Chicago. Having started dancing since the age of five years old, I have studied several styles of dance, including ballet, jazz, hip hop, and modern. When I moved to Florida in 2004, I was introduced to ballroom dancing and fell in love. Within a year, I began practicing and competing with my first partner in dance competitions all over the state, specializing in International Latin. Some of my accomplishments include placing first in my category, winning titles and scholarships at competitions such as The United States Dance Championships, Millennium Dance Sport Championships, and the Florida Superstars Dance Championships. I have also performed at the performing arts center of West Palm Beach, The Kravis Center, having been invited to dance in honor of the Kravis Board of Directors and Standing Committees, and to dance in their annual charity benefit, *Reach for the Stars*.

Ballroom dancing is my passion and has immersed me into a world full of etiquette, drive, and beauty, having taught me valuable lessons that I will forever carry with me. Reflecting on my experiences thus far in my life has motivated me to continue learning and absorbing all that I can, while also being able teach others and pass down what I have learned.

Choreology Basic

Adriana Fuentes

Hi, I am Adriana Fuentes. I was born on a hot summer day in Albuquerque, New Mexico. After my father was discharged from the Air Force, we returned to our hometown Shelton, Connecticut. This was where I had spent my early years of childhood. When I was four years old, my family relocated to South Florida. I spent my elementary years in public school, participating in various sports. I was nine years old when I started to participate in summer musical theater programs. These programs had sparked a strong interest for theater and music. Instead of going to public middle school, my parents and I decided that I would be homeschooled. Currently, I was continually becoming more involved in theatre arts. In three years, I had been in productions of *Fiddler on the Roof, God spell, The Seussical,* and *Hamlet* and was part of choirs at local schools. When I started high school, I became fully immersed in my academic studies. This limited my theatre activities.

My life unexpectedly changed in November of my junior year when I had my first ballroom lesson. At first, I did not want to participate in a ballroom dancing program for homeschoolers. When my mom told me that our family was invited to a ballroom lesson by our now close family-friends, I was far from thrilled and was against the notion of ballroom dancing when I was informed that I couldn't wear my beloved jeans. That night, my parents practically had to drag me to the ballroom, but I am so grateful that they did, or I would have never discovered the beauty of Ballroom. Since then, I have developed a strong passion and love for all the ballroom dances.

Ballroom Dancing has impacted my life in the best way possible. Firstly, ballroom has provided an opportunity for my family and me to connect and do something that we can all do together. It has also been an environment where I have made and developed friendships. In my training, I'm not only being taught 10 different and equally magnificent dances, I am also learning etiquette, how to professionally present myself, and how to teach others. As a dance instructor, I hope to do what my dance instructor was able to do with me, which was introduce ballroom as a beautiful art that

Michel F. Jacques

is significantly beneficial and can be attained by anyone. I will also be able to help others develop a love and appreciation for ballroom/Latin dance. I plan to continue my education in ballroom dancing and to dance for the remainder of my life. I am truly excited to see where my teaching certifications take me and what ballroom dancing opportunities will come knocking on my door.

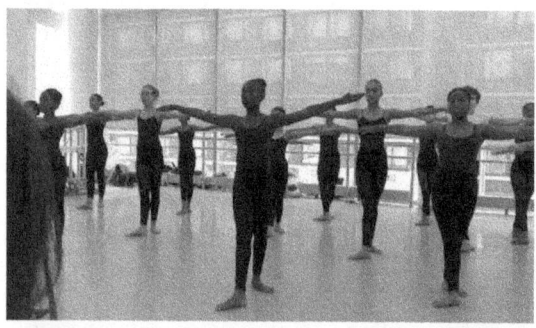

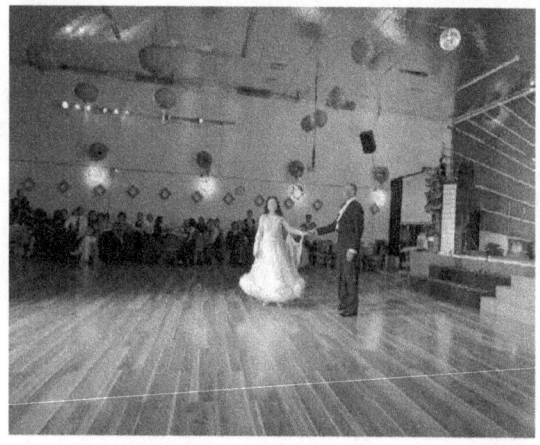

Zoltan Vincze

I am Zoltan Michael Vincze. I was born on June 21st, 1998, 9:00 PM in Danbury, Connecticut. I am blessed with a wonderful family, my parents Zoltan F. Vincze and Gabriella E. Vincze, and my younger brother Zsolt C. Vincze. Ballroom dancing was part of our lives at a young age. When I was eight years old, our parents began to take our family to ballroom dance classes. My parents have an amazing ballroom dance teacher in Connecticut who taught all of us to dance. Yours truly had a problem; he had no interest in dancing with girls. In short, I quit.

A depressing and disheartening affair took place in 2008. My whole family had an affliction know as Lyme's disease. I was so sick I couldn't continue school and was forced to quit my private school in fifth grade as a result of Lyme's. I was on homebound education from fifth grade to seventh grade. I have been home schooled since eighth grade. In 2011, my parents found a holistic healing doctor who lived in Florida. My family would drive or fly from Connecticut to Florida for treatments from him. In fact, the doctor was the reason we moved down to Florida. I battled with this auto-immune ailment from 2008 to 2012.

I had my victory against the bacteria of Lyme's disease in 2013. As I was nearing the end of my struggles with Lyme's in 2012, I decided to give ballroom another try. The first dance class I took was on October 27, 2012, where we met Francois.

In the past, I'd reminisce about the past wishing I have never quit dancing. But now, I realize it was not meant to be, at least not then. I came to Florida kicking and screaming. Now it's my favorite place in the world. I didn't enjoy dancing. Now it's my passion. I missed my old friends. Now I found my best friends. I enjoyed being in school and thought I'd never expand my mind any other way. Now, I learn more being homeschooled than I ever could in a private school. The point is, I learned to love what is now, not what was then, and to willingly follow what was planned for me by God.

My goal is...well...to be honest, I'm not quite sure. I had many goals when I lived in Connecticut, and none of them had anything to do with ballroom. My ambitions have changed countless times within the past years, and I'm only 15. Right now, I would love to be one of the best ballroom dancers in the world. When I'm dancing, it's as if the world stops, but at the same time I feel so alive. My goal as a dancer could be winning the Open level Standard Ballroom competition in Black pool, England. Afterwards, I plan on teaching dance. I might be a pro dancer on Dancing with the Stars, but I don't like contemporary and jazz, so we'll have to see. I've also always wanted to take my chances with singing, acting. I enjoy creating and starring my in-home movies, and surfing (less than a year ago, I dreamed to be a pro surfer). If one asks what my plan in life is, I would have to say I don't know, because frankly, I don't. It's all up to God. He's the one who planned my move to Florida, He's the one who gave me wonderful friends, He's the one who inspired me to dance, and most of all He's the one who gave me life. If there's anyone to ask, it's Him.

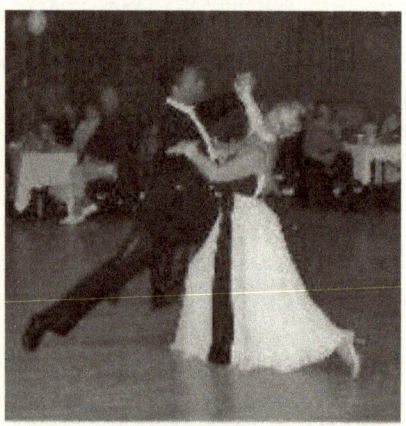

Suzanne Litwinka

Suzanne started dancing as she took her first steps. She has a passion for the dance, in any form. Her first official dance class took place in August 2001 when she was 2 years of age, but she would dance anyplace and at any time prior to that, just for the sheer joy of it!

Suzanne has studied and performed many forms of dance, including: Ballet, Pointe, Modern, Jazz, Tap, Mime, Musical Theatre, and Flamenco. Ballroom is her current focus, where she is mastering: Bolero, Cha-Cha, Fox Trot, Hustle, Meringue, Rumba, Salsa, Slow Waltz, Swing, Tango, and Viennese Waltz. Suzanne is looking forward to serving as a Certified Ballroom Dance Instructor.

In addition to dance, Suzanne has been singing with the Young Singers of the Palm Beaches since 2009. She was selected as a featured dancer for various choreographed pieces in their twice-yearly shows. Suzanne is currently a member of their Cantate choir.

Designing and creating fashions and accessories is another one of her interests. Suzanne has been sewing since 2011.

Suzanne has attended summer Theatre Arts intensive programs for the past few years where she has studied with current and former Broadway performers. A highlight for her was to work with Tony award winning choreographer, Jerry Mitchell and perform a dance number from his work in, "Hairspray".

Currently, Suzanne is a student at the prestigious Alexander W. Dreyfoos School of the Arts where she is a Theatre major. Prior to this, she had been home schooled for six years, in order to devote enough time to developing her talents in the arts.

Suzanne will continue to follow her lifelong passion for the dance as she plans her goals for the future!

Michel F. Jacques

Isabela Fuentes

Hi, my name is Isabela Veronica Fuentes. About a year ago, I started training to become a ballroom and Latin dance teacher. I am an 8th grade student at Palm Beach Virtual School. I was born in Bridgeport, Connecticut and moved to Florida when I was just a few months old. As a young girl, I spent my days playing with friends, going to parks, and enjoying the Palm Beach County weather and community. When I was around five years old, I tried out ballet and tap dancing at the local community center and didn't really take to it; I feel that it wasn't my time or style and I'm glad that my "pink princesses and ponies" personality told me to quit since ballroom is definitely the dance for me. Since then, I continue to grow in having amazement, appreciation, and respect for all music especially classical, which I find beautiful and absolutely breath taking. Ironically, I also took one Latin dancing class when I was little but at that time I wasn't interested.

When I started ballroom/Latin dancing in November 2012, I was not excited about it at all. At this point in my life, I was over the idea of dancing and didn't see the point of it but I thank God every day that my parents forced me to the first few class and my first ballroom party, where I fell in love with dancing. I remember going to the St. Patrick's Day party with my now two close friends, their parents, my sister, and my mom and I absolutely fell in love with the ballroom atmosphere, people, and style. I love ballroom dancing and hope that one day as a teacher I will inspire newcomers in the ballroom/Latin industry just as my teacher has inspired me.

Gian Di Franco

Gian Di Franco began his dance training at the age of ten at the Palms West Ballroom in Royal Palm Beach, Florida. At Palms West he was trained by the director, Herb Vazquez and a past Russian champion, Alex Foraponova. Gian began competing with his partner at age eleven. He received first place awards at many prominent ballroom competitions. He received the Top Junior award at Florida Superstars Dancesport Competition.

He went on to train with a world-renowned professional Latin couple rated 25th in the world, Andre and Natalie Paramonov. Also, this couple placed first in the world for their show dance. He trained with the Paramonovs for four years. Gian and his competitive partner received quite a few top awards at various competitions. He danced pro/am with Natalie Paramonov and placed 1st at the State Championships and 3rd in the world at Ohio Star Ball.

Gian and his partner performed shows at the Gold Coast Ballroom and had the opportunity to open the show for well-known dancers such as Karina Smirnoff, Tony Devoloni, Alex Mazo and Edyta Sliwinska, and Jose DeCamps. Gian also studied with Ivan Mulyavska and Loreta Kriksciukaityte. He received coaching from Marianne Nicole, Michael Chapman, Shirley Ballas, Paul Killick, Karina Smirnoff, and rated 4th in the world Maurizio Vescovo.

In 2011, Gian joined a dance company that made the top ten on America's Got Talent. The company performed for X-factor audience while the show was holding try-outs in Miami, FL. Also, he performed on Broadway with this company during the summer. The dance company opened for Gloria Estavan and Loniel Richie when they performed in Miami, FL.

Presently, Gian teaches with Caruso Dancesport at the Plaza Ballroom in North Palm Beach, FL. He still actively competes in international

Latin and performs in showcases with his students. He continues his training with Max Lototsky on the West Coast of FL. Eventually, he looks forward to a career as a successful professional ballroom competitor, teacher, choreographer and studio owner.

Alexandra Munoz

My name is Alexandra Marie Muñoz, and I was born on May 12, 1997. I am currently sixteen years old and am an 11th grader at Suncoast Community High School. I was born in Geneva, Illinois, outside of Chicago and lived there until the age of seven when I moved to Wellington, Florida, in 2004. I began tap, ballet, jazz, and contemporary dancing at the age of four, and competitively danced for three years in a dance troop when I was attending Okeeheelee Middle School. Eighth grade was when my interest in ballroom dancing peaked. Having been exposed to this genre of dance through my sister, Bianca, I decided to make ballroom dancing my focus.

Throughout my high school career, I have had the opportunity to continue performing and learning more about ballroom. Growing up with a Latin background, music and dance have always been very important to me and my heritage. Ballroom dancing has become an incredible part of my life and has allowed for me to fully express my love and passion for music and life.

Dominique Nemeth

My name is Dominique Nemeth. I was born on March 10, 1997 in Boca Raton Florida, and have lived here ever since! Dance has always been a significant part of my life. As I began Irish dance classes at six years old, I have literally gown up Irish dancing, and have loved every new step, every workshop, every blister and shin-splint. Ten years later, I'm still dancing, competing at the preliminary championship level and performing dozens of shows year- round. I also have found my passion for teaching dance through Irish dance and am currently working as an assistant teacher for the Rondeau School of Irish Dancing. I instruct ages four through eighteen, from the newest beginners to the more advanced competition, all nine of the traditional Irish dances as well as figures, choreographies and show dances. I also have a passion for performances and may pursue dancing with a professional dance company for a future career. I also plan on getting certified to teach Irish dance professionally, by earning my T.C.R.G, soon.

Ballroom and Latin dancing have been a completely new experience, one I never thought I would be able to participate in, but I am so thrilled that I am able to! I love being able to include my arms and upper body in the dancing as well, which is a luxury never allowed in Irish dancing. Additionally, ballroom is far more established and accepted than any other thing I've done before. I have every intention and am very eager to improve in both ballroom and Latin dancing, continuing either socially, competitively or professionally, or perhaps all three!

Thank you for your time

Choreology Basic

Dancing in Dictionary.com is Described as to move rhythmically to music, using prescribed or improvised steps and gestures. According to scriptures, the word Dance, Dances, Dancing is used over 20 times in the bible. Those words are used in the bible in two different ways.

Jumping up and down for fun to enjoy yourself. Samuel 2, verse 14—16 said that King David danced before the lord with all his might, David was wearing a linen ephod. As the ark of the lord came into the city of David, Michal, Saul's daughter looked through a window and saw King David leaping and whirling before the lord.

Exotus 15: 20-21, Miriam the prophetess led the women in dance and songs, praising God for bringing them home safe through the red sea. In a sense that men and women interacting together in a club or party jumping up and down with joy is synonym to happiness a form of celebration.

Exotus 32: Children engaging in immorality in a biblical sense, they are dancing around it. Moses Came down, he strongly condemned them for that reason. Many of us believe, every time men and women dance together it was condemned. That is not the style of Dancing I am referring to the style of dance in the night clubs. There is no passage that says, we shall not dance. However, there are some addressing dance and certain principles and the reasons why dancing is wrong.

Gallations 5: 19. When the works of a flesh are manifested adultery, formication, uncleanness, sensuality, lustful pleasure it is wrong. The Greek described those manners as filty, indecent bodily movements, unchaste handling of males and females. There are talking about men and women holding each other closely rubbing their bodies together. Dancing to suggestive music conducts which excite lust.

Gallations 5: 21. Paul said: Those who do such things shall not inherit the kingdom of God. The type of Dancers/Choreographers will not go to heaven. Those type of dancing is sinful when it involves children, young adult girls and even ladies lavishly dressed, flying up on the dance floor engaging in provocative movements sexual in nature. In fact, there is nothing wrong with having team spirit on the dance floor. It simply said the lord will keep you out of heaven. To lust for her has already committed adultery with her in his heart. Lusting for a woman who's not your wife is a sin. Since dancing is sexual in nature it is created lust.

Mark 6: 21-22 Explained it all. There were dancers engaged in suggestive bodily movements to please highly official. Herod was pleased emotionally, excited and stimulated by the dance. As a result, he made a foolish vow, something he regretted. Those type of performances are created to make people do things they would not have done in a normal life.

Dr. Rita Hollingsworth coted "Dancing is an exciting pleasurable recreation, as it affords a partial satisfaction of the sex impulse – An erotic stimulant that even works for boys & girls as young as 8 years old, even younger in many studies." The sexual nature of dancing is known all over the world. Let's stop there and go back to some of the benefits of Dance as a form of prayer, a dialogue with the architect of the universe who created us, the sky, the cosmos and everything on earth.

We have to continue our research to look at dance as a stimulator for the brain safety. What we learned and put in our heads is exactly what you get. According to science, the function of the brain is about the communication between the cells. The process of how information is stored is a highly Complex study.

My mom Macilia Saint-Paul thought me about the contents of the four parts in the human brain and how they work during our entire life. She said in my brain there are 60% human, 20% animal, 15% hates and 5% spiritual parts. What you learned and develop the most is exactly what you become to be in reality. Animals for instance are slightly different in nature. They are born with 60% animal, 20% human, 15% evils and 5% spiritual that is why they are called animals. My dad Emmanuel D. Legagneur Jacques did approve it. This helped me understand a perfect working stimulator for myself. What made us different than other human characters and animals.

I am not concern about the creation of a new brain stimulator. My focus was to conduct specific research studies on the construction and the design of human movements in Dance and its equivalence to music. I went to college and studied electrical engineering, Dance movements, Music construction, video/filmmaking and cinema. With a degree in Business ownership and Management, I was able to devote myself in managing artists Musicians and Dancers from different ethnicities and background in the United States of America as a Haitian/American and made a good living out of dancing.

For so many years working in the realm of performing arts production, I viewed Dance as a sacred and divine language. It's a true national and cultural identity which needed more attention in countries economy. It is a big responsibility, when it comes to educating our children on how to dance. Dance practitioners have to do more research on the origin of dance to compliment themselves. When we move ourselves from students to teachers, we would be able to follow policies and create respect for each other works and visions. The fact is to train and develop more dancers to become entrepreneurs and leader entrepreneurs to become dancers.

Many dance instructors around the world, especially in the Island of Haiti are teaching konpa dancing based upon their own visions on what it is. Many Countries now are in the obligation to create a standardized system on the three levels of dance education, Bronze, Silver and Gold in their own cultural music and dance art forms. The children have to have that as part of their social, cultural skills before they get to college to be able to compete in life.

I tried to be more realistic on collecting data from friends and colleagues. In the field of Ballroom and Latin social, cultural dance art forms, I recreated this elementary syllabus with easy to follow instruction to an ended result. This work allow train and certify teachers of dance to interact together, differentiate between theoretical and experimental approaches.

Michel F. Jacques

In Roman 7:1-3 talking about Lifetime marriage between Men and Women. To understand everything in the bible, according to research made by many of my colleagues, we must see all the pictures. We cannot take one verse and ignore the rest in the subject of marriage, divorce, remarried and adultery. You know, what will happen to us after death. In my dad lifetime 96 years, I presume based on statistic more than 4 million people had died on earth over his lifetime. Soon you and I will experience death and may go to Hades but, death I believe in a choreographer mind is not exist.

According to Dr. Erwin Lutzer, "God had put eternity in our head". The bible said it is appointed unto men to die once and after there will be a judgement. Jesus talk about a rich and poor man who died. Luke 16: 23-24 you see both went to Hades. But yet, both experienced different things: pain torments.

We have to understand what we see when someone die. We can see him in rest and what he is experiencing in his restless body is living in a different world. So, to speak about my experience with my dad funeral, I convinced death is not a positive experience for anyone. A need to know what happens after we die.

However, our heart is so often burst with the fullness of treasured moments in time, as we continue on this journey called life, to stop often and realize that each and every one of us has everything within to be happy and content. To be capable of inner wisdom in giving and receiving unconditionally, to count our blessings in every sight to see, in the music from high to low, what leads the body to the dance and becomes an inspiration toward keeping a healthy body and soul. Throughout the ages music and dance have been a connecting golden thread between the people of all countries. Dance has continued to nourish our soul in the direction of happiness, good health, faith and serenity. There is always and forever the joy of the music and the dance.

Choreology Basic

Many of us living a life talking about channeling, connecting with people who had died. In the mind of a choreographer death should not exist because, music, dance, peace and love are the same word poured in the bible. Let's find out what is wrong with dancing in a biblical sense. It is amazing how many songs there are with the word dance. Dancing becomes the latest primetime rage on television. Dancing is extremely popular and it is something that children have to deal with every day. What the bible said about dancing and what God think of these issues may be different. Ballroom dancing as part of the youth education starting at middle school is what I am talking about. Learning social cultural dance art forms well will lead the world to peace.

The secret ingredient is when it comes to Dance, we all need to listen to music rhythm the right way. Rhythm is a Sacred and a spiritual element within music that cannot be change. Dancing is a form of prayer, a dialogue with the architect of the Universe guides us to live an everlasting life. All rhythms came from the Cosmos and the Divine.

Dancing off timing to music is considered a misinterpretation of rhythm, leading dancers to develop lack of concentration, and respect to the artist musician who creates it. Those young dance practitioners tend to develop multiple chronic feeling disorders, stresses, lack of concentration and respect between themselves.

Aparently they would not understand and follow laws that governs nature nor nations. There are 5 key elements that fall into the construction of Music. The first one is Rhythm as specific within all the sounds that cannot be changed, It should sound the same from beginning to the end. Second is the Tempo, referred to the speed how fast and slow the music supposes to play. That's dealt to the individual brain capacity to understand. Third is Count & beats Values. Which beat in the music is the 1, the 2, the 3, and the 4. Fourth is MPM or

BPM (Measures per minute or Bar per minute). Firth is High & low created to help us identify all the beats values. Dancers should know.

Dancing is the equivalence of music. There are Universities all over the world where young adult can go for a career in music. There are not enough school yet for dance educators to get a degree. The reason why this book is written as a remedy for change toward a better world and the creation of a new dancing community.

ABOUT THE AUTHOR

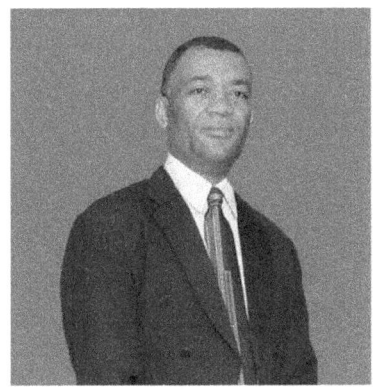

In 1984, I ventured to the United States to pursue and further develop a career in film directing. I was invited to join the Arthur Murray Board of Ballroom Dance educators in its rigorous teaching training program. My career brought me in contact with the owner of one of the largest ballroom/nightclubs in South Florida, Kays Starlite Ballroom, Inc. in Hallandale Beach, Florida. Through efforts at this establishment, I was instrumental in bringing the Haitian community together in celebration and demonstration of their ethnic and cultural unity through Konpa Dancing. I began the development of a multicultural club organization that would embrace and bring together people of all ethnic backgrounds and offered the opportunity to exchange cultural diversity through the art of ballroom dancing. I successfully founded the New Millennium Ballroom College Inc.

There are countless grammar rules in the English language. From rules on misplaced modifiers and subject/verb agreement to rules on double negatives, there are many guidelines on dictionary for us to follow when writing just about anything. However, one of the best ways to learn correct grammar is to review examples of bad grammar.

Michel F. Jacques

Choreology definition: Noun the study of the aesthetic and science of forms of human movement, movement notation. It is often called the Benesh Movement. Notation. Origin the term was coined by Rudolf and Joan Benesh in the late 40's. I had the opportunity to study from. It is an advanced techniques dealt with the graphic design of foot-point in classical dancing. Not yet available to the general public.

Dancing as a universal language is more than just movements. The interpretation of music created with notations of specific sounds dancers should study first to avoid mis-communication, bones injuries, Mental illness and chronic feeling disorders among young adults dancing under the sound of noise.

Lexico said: 'Though most widely used in ballet companies, choreology has subsequently been evolved to deal with non-classical movement also, and together with Annotation is the most internationally used system.' 'People also ask, 'Well, why do we need to have choreology, in this day and age of videotape with a question mark. Yet, there is no accurate answers. Our children must learn the difference between sound of noise and music.

I learn How to use the toe, boll, Heel in the Mambo, konpa, cha-cha-cha and the heel, boll, toe of the fox-trot, slow waltz and the tango. Konpa dancing was just a natural mores, I did not see the need to go to school to learn it. Like the Creole language I learn how to speak and make myself understood but, cannot read and write. It was a shame being forced going to school to learn how to write, read and speak foreign tongues over my own native language. It was impossible to claim a national identity, We are victim of an inter-cultural integgretion.

Contents of this version of this book choreology basic volume two is, based on various biblical research studies. Also, researches made by some of my colleagues member of CID (International Dance Council) for our readers and dance practitioners to promote diversity through Ballroom Dancing. Offering exchange of idea between professional. Looking at myself dancing to the equivalence of music help me develop a better, healthier brain stimulation. It looks like yesterday that I was a student at Policar International Dance School in Port-au-Prince, Haiti getting my first exposure to Ballroom, Social and Cultural Dance.

The use of my imagination was in 1980-1984, learning the graphic design of foot points. My work with Policar was an eye-opening in many respects. The power of thoughts both to change inappropriate habitual patterns and teach them to my students is part of my inspiration in this book.

MICHEL FRANCOIS JACQUES
Dance & Science Innovator – Choreographer, Sound engineer –Social Dance-Entrepreneur

DANCE AS A UNIVERSAL LANGUAGE

A Proactive Initiative for Dance, Health & Fitness

Francois, a legendary ballroom dance pioneer armed with an Associate of Science degree in the Business of Music and Video, is a longtime resident of the City of Hallandale establishing his first Ballroom Dance Club called Luigi's in Hallandale Beach in 1992.

In 2007, while pursuing a Bachelors of Arts in Filmmaking at the Art Institute of Fort-Lauderdale, Francois joined The International Association for Dance Medicine and Science. This union with IADMS inspired Francois to create yet another ground-breaking business venture resulting from his extensive travels and research study of Dance in Greece, Germany, England, Japan, Europe, India and Central & South America. Fast-Forward 5 years and the dance icon returns to the scene with a revolutionary concept to create a one-stop-shop Dance Studio & Wellness Center franchise.

Michel F. Jacques

The overall purpose of New Millennium Health Services was to meet the individual needs of clients to assure that they receive the TOTAL WELLNESS EXPERIENCE. In addition to the dance professionals the facility was also catered to families, children, corporations (public and private) who are seeking to explore a NEW approach to Dance Fitness and Wellness that enables them to immerse their body, mind, and spirit into a new life style that celebrates the complete maximization of their truest potential" says Francois.

Francois is a true architect of human movement. His zealous passion to educate, communicate and promote true cultural awareness is a fresh perspective that is more than just analyzing the posture of whether one is standing or sitting correctly but moreover the expression of how movement is the connective force that celebrates the true sense of genetic and cultural heritage.

1) Michel Francois Jacques is now President of the Hallandale Section of CID UNESCO Inc.

2) Active member of: IADMS (International Association for Dance medicine & Science)

- **HEALING THROUGH MOVEMENT**
- **"RESTORING THE FOUNDATIONS OF OUR SOUL**
- **<u>Section I:</u>** How our brain functions with regards to Movement in the Healing Process
- **<u>Section II:</u>** Activating the Principles

Choreology Basic

HOW OUR BRAIN FUNCTIONS WITH REGARDS TO MOVEMENT IN THE HEALING PROCESS

Throughout history and Biblical history, movement and specifically dance movement has been associated with:

- Joy
- Thanksgiving
- Victory
- Triumph

HEALING SYNCHRONIZED MOVEMENT

Two examples of truths concerning ourselves personally and as a group of people in unity, expressing healing synchronized movement:

- **Psalms 30:11** "Thou hast turned for me my mourning into dancing: thou hast put off my sackcloth, and girded me with gladness;"
- **Jeremiah 31:13** "Then shall the virgin rejoice in the dance, both young men and old together: for I will turn their mourning into joy, and will comfort them, and make them rejoice from their sorrow."

OUR BRAIN AND HOW IT FUNCTIONS

- **<u>Front Part of OUR Brain:</u>**
- Associated with Social Skills
- Desire
- Personal Preference
- Our Identity
- **<u>Back Part of OUR Brain:</u>**
- Associated with Stored Memories
- Feelings that hold us captive

    God wants us to live in peace with a synchronized brain.

We respond and function out of what we have learned. We can re-pattern our experiences through movement.

THE SYNCHRONICITY OF HEALING MOVEMENT

In 1950 the word ***Synchronicity*** was coined by Carl Jung a psychologist of human behavior. It came out of a study of one of his patients who could not assimilate rational truth with her own inner consciousness.

- **<u>Synchronicity</u>:** when things happen together, as if perfectly timed.

In movement not only is the front and back parts of our brain engaged; but also the right and left hemispheres.

- **<u>Right Hemisphere</u>**: Experiential
- **<u>Left Hemisphere</u>:** Language and Descriptions

When our knowledge doesn't mirror our experiences, the depth of our understanding is hindered.

RE-PATTERNING EXPERIENCES THROUGH MOVEMENT

Synchronized movement alternating between hemispheres helps to bring this meshing of knowledge and experience, bringing balance to our brains and bodies.

<u>Body Memories:</u>
- Our bodies hold memories which can lead to different illnesses. As we move, becoming more connected to the divine personally, we can choose to release the trauma of stored memories and allow our bodies to heal themselves on that level.

- A good resource: "The most excellent way" <u>www.tmewcf.org</u>

RE-PATTERNING EXPERIENCES THROUGH MOVEMENT

Dance synchronizes our brains bringing the left and right sides together. When your brain is synchronized it brings you into a state of joy. Endorphins are released which bring healing and peace to our spirits. When we are in joy we have great capacity to deal with the trauma in our lives. We receive this joy when we become synchronized within ourselves and with others. Joy allows you to be open and transparent. Joy brings a quietness and peace to your body; healing the restless soul.

JOY IS CONTAGIOUS

SYNCHRONIZED UNITY: SPIRIT, SOUL AND BODY

Shalom (Peace) is achieved through synchronization.
Meaning: nothing broken, nothing divided.
Some of the Benefits of Movement:

- Strengthens our Lungs
- Improves Posture, Grace and Agility
- Increases Bone Density
- Improves our Balance and Builds Muscles
- Aids in Weight Loss and Improves Confidence
- Releases Endorphins

PUTTING ON THE GARMENT OF PRAISE

It has been medically proven that laughter, joy, touch, and affirmation are all ingredients for healing of our physical bodies. Most of the time it is a decision we must make for our own well being first. As we receive our healing we are able to bring others along the same path.

- "Freedom is found in Movement" ***John Paul Jackson***
- "Put on the garment of Praise for the Spirit of heaviness" ***Isaiah 61:3***

Michel F. Jacques

THE SACRED DANCE OF CREATION

Movement is intrinsic to all things created. Everything is in motion; the seen and unseen. We were created to move. Some of us are comfortable with choreographed pieces and some free style, spontaneous or prophetic dance. Whatever style you embrace, let your creativity be released for yourself and others who may be touched by what they see and experience.

THE LAW OF RESONANT FREQUENCY

The author of "The Energetic Heart," Rollin McCraty, Ph.D. explains the heart, like the brain, generates a powerful electromagnetic field, only much larger. He says, "The heart generates the largest electromagnetic field in the body. The electrical field as measured in an electrocardiogram (ECG) is about 60 times greater in amplitude than the brain waves recorded in an electroencephalogram (EEG). So we see God created us with the capacity to communicate at levels much deeper than verbal communication, one of those being "cardio-gnosis" (heart to heart knowledge)

DANCING TOGETHER

Partnering with someone else in the dance or in spontaneous movement brings another dimension to the healing process. Mirroring movements with a partner can also build synchronicity in both people and an endorphin called Oxytocin is released. This particular endorphin actually has been shown to produce trust among the partners. Trust is a chief component in the healing process; no matter by whatever means or paths we choose for the purpose of healing.

It is our highest goal to live a full productive life. Enjoying ourselves, each other, creation and experiences shared. Movement on any level can help us achieve these desires. Dance is one of the many enjoyable ways to achieve this. As we move, we heal, but as we dance we release the added component of joy we experience to others

By: Karen Simmons

- **Teaching Seminars**
- **Prophetic Intercession Seminars**
  Spiritual Mapping Seminars

- *Inner Court Ministries*
- "Serving the Body of Christ since 1987"
  Founder and Director: Karen Simmons
  www.innercourtministries.org

www.ingramcontent.com/pod-product-compliance
Lightning Source LLC
Chambersburg PA
CBHW031157020426
42333CB00013B/703